Feeding EDEN

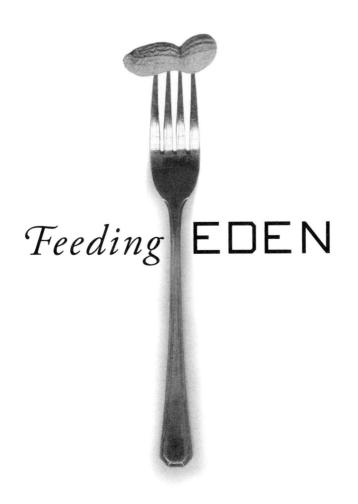

Feeding EDEN

THE TRIALS AND TRIUMPHS OF A FOOD ALLERGY FAMILY

SUSAN WEISSMAN

STERLING
New York

For my family – Drew, Dayna, and Eden

STERLING
New York

An Imprint of Sterling Publishing
387 Park Avenue South
New York, NY 10016

ISBN 978–1-4027–8122–3 (hardcover)
ISBN 978–1-4027–8969–4 (ebook)

Distributed in Canada by Sterling Publishing
^c/o Canadian Manda Group, 165 Dufferin Street
Toronto, Ontario, Canada M6K 3H6
Distributed in the United Kingdom by GMC Distribution Services
Castle Place, 166 High Street, Lewes, East Sussex, England BN7 1XU
Distributed in Australia by Capricorn Link (Australia) Pty. Ltd.
P.O. Box 704, Windsor, NSW 2756, Australia

For information about custom editions, special sales, and premium and corporate purchases, please contact Sterling Special Sales at 800–805–5489 or specialsales@sterlingpublishing.com.

Manufactured in the United States of America

2 4 6 8 10 9 7 5 3 1

www.sterlingpublishing.com

CONTENTS

FOREWORD

AN ALLERGIST'S WAITING ROOM IS THE first support group for most allergy families. When I began practicing thirty-five years ago, I heard snatches of conversation in our waiting room that were wiser than much of what I told parents about coping with their children's conditions. Also, little things I had told a mother (it is usually the mother) years before would find their way to a mom whose child was new to treatment. It made me a better doctor. Hoping to harness this resource, thirty years ago we started a support group, and it has been going on ever since; for the past twenty years it has been under the hand of Kathy Franklin. Kathy and I both appear in this book—she by name; I am identified only as "our attending physician."

Allergic diseases are mysterious. They arise when part of the immune system that has evolved to attack parasites instead goes after proteins in otherwise harmless items such as pollens and peanuts, which Susan's son is allergic to, along with other foods. Allergies and asthma have been recognized for thousands of years. (Among other delights, Susan goes on informative tangents to explain things like this history.) But for about the past forty years, the incidence has grown geometrically, first with nasal allergies like those to pollen, then asthma, and more recently, food allergy. We don't know why, although the way we live and eat, climate change, and medical treatment are all implicated. Regardless, we haven't caught up with the epidemic, medically or socially. Current medical literature recounts exciting research that, if proven, is still years away from providing effective treatment. Other research shows how badly we are doing at utilizing current best practices. For example, only around half of asthmatics are treated according to established guidelines, and even those receiving recommended treatment fail to comply about half the time.

The numbers for food allergy are smaller than for asthma, but the feelings are more intense. Food allergies are someone else's problem until they are *your* problem, and then they become all-consuming. As I have observed in my practice, food allergy is the fulcrum for unbalancing all kinds of family behavior: parents blame one another, in-laws resent in-laws, grandparents make mistakes and tempt fate by feeding children forbidden foods with unconditional love, siblings feel left out, and so on.

Peanuts are a lightning rod because of their role in the standard child's diet. The low point came early in 2011 when a Florida six-year-old was driven out of her public school by parents who resented restrictions on their own children's behavior. These are unreasonable times, and peanut allergies seem to inflame passions that mimic other societal fault lines. I tell parents not to be bashful about protecting their children because "they" don't understand—"they" being those who don't send the kids off to school wondering if there might be a medical emergency later in the day from something innocuous to most of us. How could something as ordinary as peanut butter be toxic? On the other hand, I do not agree with some of the most restrictive ideas out there.

I have always felt that the movement to educate "them" would be well served by eavesdropping on our waiting room and support group chat, which combines, by turn, naiveté among the newcomers and knowledge from the veterans, helplessness and can-do spirit, despair and humor. Feeding Eden brings all that together. For all the stories I have heard, all the mothers I have listened to, I have never gotten so thoroughly into the experience of a child, the effects on a marriage and a sibling, and above all the mind of a mom as I do with the Weissmans when Susan throws herself into the unexpected health challenges of her adored son.

Susan also holds a mirror up to medicine (and alternative medicine) in ways that ought to give all of us pause. Among the many strengths of this book is the way Susan describes her frustration with a succession of practitioners, necessitating her acquisition of the skills and knowledge to evaluate the care Eden had been getting both inside and outside the medical mainstream. This is a journey that many others have embarked on and many more unsuspecting parents will have to take. They will all benefit by reading this book.

—Dr. Paul M. Erhlich

Dr. Paul M. Ehrlich is a partner at Allergy and Asthma Associates of Murray Hill in Manhattan, clinical assistant professor of pediatrics at New York University School of Medicine, coauthor of Asthma Allergies Children: A Parent's Guide, *and cofounder of AsthmaAllergiesChildren.com. He is a fellow of the American Academy of Pediatrics; the American Academy of Allergy, Asthma & Immunology; and the American College of Allergy, Asthma & Immunology; and president of the New York Allergy and Asthma Society. He has been featured as one New York's top pediatric allergists in* New York *magazine for more than a decade.*

INTRODUCTION: CRAZY

THE JANUARY SKY SHED WAFERS OF SNOW onto our coats during the short walk home. By the time we reached our building on East 87th Street in New York City, the descent had quickened. My four-year-old child, Dayna, and I pulled at our watery boots outside the front door of our apartment while she offered a detailed report on yet another birthday party. Too full of pink frosting and sugar doughnuts, she decided to forgo lunch and hurried off to her dollhouse as if an event had begun without her. I headed straight for the kitchen, where I saw my younger child, one-year-old Eden, fussing, his faint eyebrows knitted vigorously. My mother-in-law, Eden's "Nana," who had baby-sat for the last hour, announced as soon as she saw me, "He needs to eat. But I waited." As she hurried him into his high chair, I imagined her anxiously eyeing the covered bowl on the counter, suffering the slow minutes I was out.

It was getting harder to watch Eden eat these days, even for me, and so instead of hovering over his tufted round head, I decided to use the time to sort through my designated drawer, which was comfortably close in the adjoining dining room. Whereas the top drawer of the credenza was reserved for Eden's stroller enhancements such as key chains and scraps of Velcro, and the middle drawer was for the generic junk of my husband, Drew—checkbooks, wallets, keys, eyeglasses—mine was more revealing and held subtle clues to my current life. There were handwritten notes of phone conversations with Eden's doctors, old unsorted photos, half-squeezed tubes of Eden's rejected skin lotions, an invitation to a come-and-gone alumni event, a sparkly hair elastic purchased for Dayna that I kept forgetting about, and a flyer from a United Jewish Appeal Women's Committee that I kept without any intention of joining but which served as a warning that I might be in danger of becoming one of those mothers who are all about their children—or child.

I was only a few feet behind Eden's high chair, clutching handfuls of paper, when Nana called out to me, "He's scratching his neck."

Before I could turn and walk the three feet of wooden floor, she added with uncharacteristic insistence, "Susan! Susan, look *now*. He's *really* scratching his neck."

Eden wasn't so much scratching his neck as clawing at it. His nail streaks had raised red flesh. Above them, one cheek was oddly lumpy, as if he were a squirrel storing food. He began to cry as I reached down and unstrapped him.

"What is it? What was it? He was fine . . . he was fine, wasn't he?" Nana asked.

I pitched my words over hers: "Nothing! What could it be? The doctor said because of his vomiting and that stupid milk thing we did, we should just stick with lamb and rice or maybe bananas . . . that's what's in the bowl . . . that was it . . . rice and lamb. What *could* it be?"

Nana silently blinked her questions at me as I paced the parquet. "I'll call the doctor—where's the phone? What's the matter, Baby? Okay, no more, no more, I'm calling . . . Yes, hello?"

As I was explaining his symptoms, the phone crooked under my neck, Eden's forearms started flushing. I got off the phone and put a syringe of Benadryl in Eden's mouth as Doctor Bennet had just suggested. It didn't help. It was supposed to slow it, but suddenly Eden's hands were puffing like two tiny baseball mitts. While I picked up the phone to call Doctor Bennet again, Eden's other cheek expanded into equilibrium. Doctor Bennet ordered, "Don't wait."

Eden was wailing as I tossed his navy coat over his back. He pawed at himself harder, more. He couldn't get at it. He couldn't satisfy the itch. I ordered my mother-in-law to call my husband at his office, and after she hustled Dayna into her bedroom and out of the way, Eden and I were in a taxi to the Lenox Hill Hospital emergency room. In the backseat Eden panted slightly. When I pulled up his shirt, his stomach was decorated with patches of rounded rectangles and smaller circles and streaks, a random topographical skin mosaic. As Eden's eyelid started swelling and his lips inflated, I was already on autopilot, running through a tunnel of panic into the hospital.

We were lucky.

The doctor said we were lucky because the emergency room was practically empty that day. "So unusual . . . Things were slow this morning . . . Maybe the weather . . . This way, this way." No stretchers racing down long halls, as I might have imagined, just walking fast and carrying Eden into a white partitioned area. There, Eden's red-and-white body was stripped, flipped, and reflipped, and then shot with liquid epinephrine.

And then the exquisite pale pink of Eden's relief after the epinephrine took effect. Everywhere his flesh seemed to exhale. Those soft hues whispered into me like warm mist: *he's safe*. Then it was quiet. He needed to rest.

I was sitting on the side of the bed, Eden's head cupped in the crook of my arm, when the doctor came back with his clipboard. He asked me questions. It seemed so important to try to keep that beautiful calm inside our space, so at first I practically whispered about Eden, about how I hadn't been able to produce enough breast milk to sustain him and had fed Eden a formula, which he had vomited for months after he was born. It wasn't until a specialist, a pediatric gastroenterologist (GI), diagnosed Eden as allergic to his milk-based formula that we understood he had an allergy. But wait. Then, a few months later, the same doctor suggested that we find out if Eden had outgrown his allergy. So just a few weeks before Eden's first birthday, I fed him some dairy foods and it didn't go well. He had been vomiting regularly ever since.

Louder now, I continued. But there wasn't any dairy in Eden's lunch. Eden's GI had cautioned me to feed him digestible foods such as ground rice and lamb. Those foods were supposed to settle his stomach, to restore him. Not do this. "What *was* this?" I asked.

I'm sure that the doctor answered me, but I don't remember exactly how he responded. I remember what he said later. Later, Eden and I were waiting to be checked out and I was thinking about Nana back at home and her split-screen images of that day—her grandson inflating from all angles while her granddaughter busily ruled the geopolitics of her dollhouse miniatures. The doctor spotted me in the hard plastic chair, silently staring out, clutching Eden, and he beamed at us. "If I might offer you some advice . . ." He looked pleased because he just saved my son's life, yes? He looked so pleased that it took a minute before I realized he was telling me an anecdote about his first child's health problem.

His opening: "My mother always used to say, you act like a meshuggener, they'll act like a meshuggener."

I'm a Jewish New Yorker and know my tribe's vernacular. *Meshuggener* is the Yiddish word for "crazy"—not the clinically insane kind of crazy, more like the hyper wild-child kind of crazy. As he spoke, the doctor's face gleamed with confidence in his advice.

And so my lifesaving emergency room doctor moved on from this introduction to tell me, in far more words, that he and his wife had been a bit overprotective of their first daughter when she had a little colic. But the real problem was that they continued their solicitous and slightly crazy behavior even after their baby girl was long over said colic. As a result, he believed, his daughter became demanding and capricious, causing his mother to ask them why their little one always acted so crazy. That was when he and his wife had their epiphany about modeling behaviors for their child.

He finished his story with these lines: "So, just because you've been to the emergency room, you don't want a meshuggener on your hands later. Don't let his allergies make you crazy."

Here's what I think. I think the emergency room doctor, who had probably seen more than his share of it, surely didn't want me to go forth feeling crazy. But in fact, according to the Asthma and Allergy Foundation of America, food allergies account for 30,000 visits to the emergency room each year.[1]

Crazy. But did that doctor have any idea how crazy Eden's allergies seemed? He wrote Eden's diagnosis simply: anaphylaxis. Cause unknown. Anaphylaxis is defined as a "a serious allergic reaction that is rapid in onset and may cause death," and you need to have only one of these sets of symptoms to be diagnosed with anaphylaxis: the first, skin symptoms (such as hives or swollen lips) and either difficulty breathing *or* signs of low blood pressure; the second is possible exposure to a suspected allergen plus two or more of the following: breathing problems, skin symptoms of any kind, low blood pressure, and symptoms affecting the gut (such as vomiting or cramping); the third, exposure to a known allergen *and* signs of low blood pressure.

The trigger for Eden's anaphylactic reaction that day was never identified. Most likely, it was caused by an allergy to something in his lunch. The possibilities ranged widely:

1. I had unwittingly used a dairy-free margarine that contained "soy protein isolate" and Eden, we would learn later, was allergic to soy.
2. There were traces of butter, a dairy food, on the surface of my frying pan or other cooking utensil.
3. There were traces of something besides lamb in the ground lamb.
4. Eden had a lamb or rice allergy, both of which are uncommon (disproved after testing).
5. Eden reacted to the combined exposure of the margarine containing soy, possible trace amounts of butter tainting the frying pan, and/or other unidentified proteins contained in the ground lamb.

The possibilities may not have been endless, but within a week of that visit Eden's allergies seemed that way. Could the ER doctor have foreseen that we would go to an allergist who would perform skin, blood, and urine tests and pronounce Eden allergic to soy, eggs, dairy, tree nuts, peanuts, beans, fish, shellfish, plums, peaches, and cherries? If he had known about Eden's long list of foods, would he still have told me not to be crazy?

What if that same doctor knew that in four years we would intrepidly visit a new peanut-free diner that opened in our neighborhood and witness one of Eden's worst reactions? We didn't know that Eden's French fries had swum in a vat of oil with some buttermilk-coated chicken. Those fries were such a rare treat, so authentic and crispy, that even after his bottom lip swelled out like a saucer, Eden tried to keep eating for a few frenzied minutes until we pulled them away. Two minutes later, after his first dose of Benadryl, as I was pulling on my jacket, EpiPen poised, Eden's head rolled forward toward the shiny red diner tabletop. But he was just exhausted, thank God, not faint.

Would the famed spilled coffee afternoon have changed that doctor's mind? My anguished babysitter dripped three measly drops, at most, out of her lukewarm coffee cup and rinsed it all off Eden's arm before continuing on to his Tae Kwan Do class. It was Eden's turn to get a new stripe on his belt that day. But as his eyes began watering during the sparring exercises, she panicked and broke into a rare jog back to our apartment. When they burst inside, Eden's hives were growing upward out of his starchy karate uniform and into his right ear. One hour and one dose of Benadryl later, Eden got up off the couch and asked me, "Can we go back now? I want my new belt."

How wouldn't I know Crazy? Let me count the ways. Despite the doctor's counsel, Crazy and I became as intimate as lovers. Crazy became my stalker, my unwelcome houseguest, and even my muse. I see Crazy in the shadows of other parents, the parents with children like Eden. When I try to tout my sanity to teachers and friends—"Oh, and I try not to get too crazy"—Crazy laughs its ass off in the corner and continues to flit and fly all around.

After that day in the emergency room, Drew took Crazy everywhere too. He has brought Crazy to work, even to board meetings, the image of Eden's haggard eyes or rasping breaths remaining with him long after he closes our front door. Even our "well child," Dayna, has caught more glimpses of Crazy than we ever wanted. Just a few months ago, the three of us stopped off at a prepared foods store on the walk home from school. I shopped there so often that the owner, Lorenzo, knew all of us. Of course I asked twice about the potato Eden and Dayna wanted, and Lorenzo assured us that the potato was just potato. All of us heard him. So at first I didn't fully believe Eden when he pushed his plate away and repeated with a six-year-old's insistence that "something is in that potato."

Half an hour later when his wheezing began and his hives sprouted, I believed him. Dayna's eyes went wide as I pulled off Eden's shirt and guided him to the couch, away from any mirrors. That night Dayna squeezed herself in between Crazy and Eden on our red sofa while I rubbed cortisone and ice on his torso and dosed him with Benadryl and ice water. Dayna wouldn't acknowledge his swollen body and face as she challenged Eden to endless rounds on their handheld electronic game. In fact, Dayna stood up to Crazy better than any of us. Except for Eden.

Drew and I know that Crazy is our Achilles' heel: we have a child whose illness, since his eczema is under control, is rarely visible. Worse, food allergies are sometimes stigmatized at every level, from the school cafeteria to the mass media. We cringe every time we read or hear a media pun on allergies and nuts. I am perpetually surprised at how much energy I use explaining to new camp counselors, teachers, and other parents what we must do to keep Eden safe. Alive.

Before that trip to the emergency room, I looked forward. *When she is in grade school, in a few years when we travel more.* But after the emergency room, I began mothering in circles. During the upward loops, I was certain I had Eden's allergies under control. "This is it," I would reason with myself before finessing my latest strategy with Drew. "I know what to do for him so we can all feel normal again." Every time one of Eden's doctors reevaluated his diagnosis, tweaked his list of forbidden foods, offered up a new course of treatment for living with his life-threatening allergies, I would edit the narrative of our lives. Anaphylaxis? We'll tote an EpiPen! Feeding therapy? Uhh, sure! Cross-contamination? I'll make food from scratch! Asthma? Let's get inhalers! Okay. Now can we go back to our normal life?

Crazy is the hairbreadth between health and illness, intimacy and pretense, festivity and panic. With every blunder, every significant allergic reaction, my brain catapults back to the emergency room where Eden showed me how he might look before he dies. The precipice. Sometimes the mere suggestion of an accident—"Hon? Would you look at his eye? Was that kid over there eating peanut butter?"—was enough to freeze my thoughts in the middle of a crowded playground. Those were the downward curves, my numbing vision of a life with maximum safety and little joy.

And now, seven years after I met that doctor, Crazy still tries to distract me from building our big and beautiful life, one that embraces Eden's allergies. But I stay focused. Everyone else can blow off Crazy with the same tiring assumptions: "But they outgrow it, right?" or "Surely they will find a cure." Most people want to hear promises.

Now, of course I want Eden to outgrow a condition that offers him a swift and potentially unpredictable death. Of course I want him to outgrow it all: his multiple food allergies and then the asthma he developed when he was three. I want Eden to have a cure. But in the meantime, I live with Crazy, and it won't let me tell tales of deflective optimism. Instead, like many other parents, I've educated myself about my child's medical condition to find ways to live with it. I've joined a larger community of individuals and organizations devoted to developing a body of knowledge about food allergies.

As I search for my own solutions for Eden, time is on my side. There has been a statistical rise in children with food allergies and a responsive groundswell of resources, products, and general awareness. As for the parents surfing this wave together, once in a while one of us falters; we slip up. We might forget the medicine just when they need it most or fail to notice the other, nonallergic child. Often we read a label too quickly or simply buckle under the sheer effort of constant vigilance. Sometimes one of us loses pace and gets caught in his or her own undertow of despair. When that happens to me, I pull myself back up to tell the tale. So I've written what I know. Though I learn more about allergies every day, I know how life is when food makes you feel crazy.

Chapter 1

SEARCHING FOR A SAVIOR

WHEN I WAS ELEVEN YEARS OLD, my brother, Charlie, and I got *Pong*, an early television video game. The gift was a huge concession from parents who believed television taxed young eyes and minds. Although we did have a smallish TV in the family room, viewing was strictly supervised: one shared hour a night. On weekends the scheduling of *Love Boat* immediately after *Fantasy Island* caused no small measure of duress. How to choose?

Then we got lucky. Somehow Charlie convinced my parents that *Pong* was a game, not television. (My father on games for children: "When I was a kid in Brooklyn, we played stickball in the street all day. We were always playing games.") Somehow Charlie's angle worked despite the fact that *Pong* would take us not to the streets but to the screen. And we loved it; the tiny yellow ball moving in morbidly slow motion against the dark background like an ailing firefly enthralled us for many afternoons. The first two years of Eden's life I became that—a *Pong* ball bouncing foolishly and incessantly to and fro between doctors. Why? Eden's life began with vomit. It seemed like endless streams. He was born in late December, and by March my stomach clenched just thinking about his next bottle of formula. Hold his head an inch too low. Vomit. Tilt him back up one minute too soon. Vomit. Your best friend just had a new rug delivered? Vomit. Borrowing your brother's newborn glider? Vomit.

Eden didn't spit up sweet baby burps on our shoulders. He released projectile and warm liquid. An extra centimeter of forward trajectory after his bottle could empty him with the ease of ice water splashing from a ceramic pitcher on a summer day. Of course, my older child, Dayna, used to leave small gray stains on my black T-shirts and had her share of storyworthy restaurant and airplane episodes. (Nothing screams *parent* like the trading of vomit anecdotes at cocktail parties.) But Eden's vomits often filled our towels and soaked our shirts.

After three months of alternating vomit, reprieve, and then a return to Eden's bounty, I no longer could convince myself that this was nothing to be concerned about. Instead of phoning in again, I brought Eden to my pediatrician for a consultation. She was part of a bustling practice, and the waiting room was bursting with strollers and clamor, baggy-eyed mothers in velvet sweatpants, and leggy little girls jumping around an air hockey table. I watched the plastic puck skid and bounce while Eden's dozing eyelids fluttered. But after the long wait and despite my growing concern, my pediatrician believed that nothing was wrong. She wasn't worried because Eden was still on his "weight curve." It seemed his weight curve indicated that, although he was a small child, Eden was gaining weight at an appropriate rate, despite his daily purges. No red flags here.

Drew had suggested that Eden might be allergic to his formula, but when I asked about this, the pediatrician told me I was welcome to give him a soy-based formula but she doubted it would help. "It has nothing to do with the formula, you feed him. This is *normal* acid reflux, and it is *very* common."

Then she asserted that although infantile acid reflux was inconvenient, it wasn't physically or emotionally harmful to the child. I sensed her focus had shifted to her waiting room, to the pimply faced boys and frizzy-haired girls with fevers, strep infections, and lice. After our brief conversation, she wanted to move on. We all know that feeling, the sense that the doctor is done with us even though we haven't even begun to form the first question that might address our lingering uncertainties and fears.

After returning home and settling Eden down for a nap, I looked up acid reflux on the Mayo Clinic website. I learned that there is a ring of muscle between the esophagus and the stomach that must develop to prevent stomach contents from going back up into the esophagus. The website reassured me, "Most babies who have infant acid reflux are healthy."[2]

Shortly after that dreary March appointment, the air in New York began to smell green again. Mild breezes stirred around my bare hands when I strolled with Eden and, in tow, Dayna standing importantly on her toddler kickboard. Normally I love warm weather. I embrace the end of every New York winter, even knowing that the urban warmth is a harbinger of summer humidity. But that spring brought Eden rashes. Hard red pimples began creeping out from the back of his knees and then marched outward to his ankles, feet, face, arms, and legs like an army of ants. The skin on the back of his neck began peeling like old wallpaper. Bad eczema, my babysitter suggested. "My sons had it bad too."

Like many parents confronting a health issue for the first time, I took comfort in my babysitter's recognition of Eden's skin ailment. But another mother's familiarity is not as assuring as one's own. Dayna was born with a translucent olive complexion that resisted irritation, flaking, and flushes, but Eden's pallor was bumpy, chafed, and swollen all at once. As April became May, there were endless combinations of these adornments. Eden's eczema had personality, versatility. It "wept" sometimes with sticky pus.

After prescribing a cream that did nothing, my pediatrician referred me to a dermatologist named Doctor Weiss. Unfortunately, Doctor Weiss had a busy practice and the first appointment we could get was weeks away. In the interim I prowled around for my own solutions. I paced the aisles of drugstores and patted Eden down with an entire bathroom cabinet's worth of nonprescription lotions. I ordered a remedy from New Zealand that was based on rarefied bee pollen while Drew looked approvingly over my shoulder at the computer screen. "Whatever it takes!" he affirmed. He used the same phrase negotiating business deals over the phone, and I paused for a moment at his current application. But we were a team. I added oils and oatmeal into Eden's little plastic bathtub, and he emerged slick, red, and bumpy. He would look up at me and paw at himself. Constantly.

I bought soy-based formula, hoping it would solve both of Eden's issues—eczema and reflux—but after about ten days of second-guessing improvement on both fronts, it was obvious that nothing had changed. So for consistency's sake I began feeding Eden his milk formula again.

"Is the baby sleeping through the night yet?" asked our neighbor, a semiretired grandmother sporting thick glasses and a rotating wardrobe of denim A-line dresses. I threw my head back and laughed wildly: You foolish, foolish fool! Mmm, no. I collapsed at her feet. No. I smiled politely and chirped, "Not yet. Soon, for sure!" thinking of the frictionless crib sheets Drew had happened on in a catalog.

One night, after weeks of hourly sleep interruption, I heard something through my sleep. A car growled. No. Dayna called to me from a park bench. Then it was an alarm and then a howling beast or maybe a parade, with crowds of people shouting out. Then only one person was calling: a baby. He must be hurt. Whose baby? Is there a baby somewhere? *Oh, my God, how long has he been crying?* I flipped my blanket, ran through our hallway with my arms in front of me for fear of slamming my face into a wall, and reached for the screaming bump in the crib in the dark living room. "Oh, God, I'm so sorry, so sorry, so sorry," I repeated, cradling Eden as he scratched. I felt like the nightmare, the monster in my own dreams.

Finally, it was the day of our appointment with Doctor Weiss, pediatric dermatologist. When we arrived, I stared surreptitiously at the other children in his waiting room, looking for their rashes. *Did he cure them?* Next, it was all pleasant handshakes, but once in the exam room, Doctor Weiss turned on me. Literally. One hand on Eden's torso, he twisted to face me. "Your son is *normal*! This is normal eczema. Were you told otherwise?!"

I balked. I stammered. I was thirty-five years old and yet Doctor Weiss was my high school trigonometry tutor, the one with Sanka-laced breath who had scolded me at every session: "You can't learn if you're not prepared! You must prepare! Where are your flash cards?" I never had an answer to that question.

But I had an answer for Doctor Weiss. Questions too! I replied, "Well, I'm here because my pediatrician gave me a cream but it didn't work. And I have some questions." I added: "Since he's five months old, do you have any special recommendations or concerns about introducing solid food into Eden's diet . . . after seeing his skin?"

"I don't! He should be eating. Everything! He's normal! Your son should eat everything."

Suddenly my beloved Brighton Beach grandmother was in the room. Even at ten in the morning, her kosher Empire chicken was always warm from the oven and ready for carving. She used to stare at me unwaveringly, nodding and bobbing her head with approval, ensuring that I didn't miss a morsel as I ate the salty meat off the bone. "Everything!" she would exclaim, her bright blue eyes snapping happily. "Have everything. You want more?" By meal's end I would practically slip off the Formica chair in her kitchen, too full to hold myself up to the waxed tablecloth surface.

And so, armed with Doctor Weiss's experienced counsel and after four months of age-appropriate feeding, two prescription ointments, and one bottle of Zyrtec, Eden turned nine months old. He had been vomiting for exactly seven of those months. The math didn't look good. Neither did his rashes—red on red. So I took Eden to a second specialist—a pediatric gastroenterologist named Doctor Bennet. Or as my mother exclaimed later, "A stomach doctor just for children? Huh!"

And it turned out, it *did* matter what Eden ate and drank—or didn't. Five years later, in 2008, the American Academy of Pediatrics (AAP) would come to define Eden as "an infant at risk." From the year Eden was born, the definition of *at risk* was redefined from "an infant with both parents, or one parent plus a sibling with allergies" to "an infant with at least one parent or sibling with an allergic disease." That was Eden, since Drew has had kick-ass hay fever since early childhood. Drew freebased nasal steroids for years.

And me? Well, I've never had hay fever, but I had had a one-time childhood food allergy that didn't seem relevant. More important, I had bouts of viral asthma in my twenties and thirties. But guess what? If you had asked me when Eden was born if I presented a genetic risk for allergies, I would have answered, "No, I don't really have allergies." I didn't know that asthma is viewed as an associated allergic disorder with Eden's food allergies and eczema. I didn't even know the term *viral asthma*. I just knew that most of my bad colds turned into hacking coughs for which I sometimes medicated myself with prescribed bronchial inhalers.

The 2008 AAP report went on to say that for at-risk infants who are not breast-fed, there is evidence that atopic dermatitis may be delayed or prevented by giving a hypoallergenic formula.[3] Again, although I nursed Eden for about a month after his birth, a lactation consultant had determined that I wasn't able to produce enough breast milk for him to have nutritional benefits, and so he had been completely reliant on formula since that time. And I had unwittingly given him a milk protein–

based formula and a soy-based formula, neither of which is recommended by the AAP for infants with Eden's family history.

Sitting in Doctor Bennet's office, all I knew was that like any parent living with that much vomit and pus, a mother whose house was covered in protective bath towels that draped the furniture like lazy Renoir women, I wanted to make it stop. Maybe that's why I brushed off his very first question to me: "Do *you* vomit your food?"

Doctor Bennet asked it quietly. Did he ask all his patients' parents this question? Standard? Minutes before his inquiry, I had stood in his hallway with Eden's belly pressed against me and read the doctor's mural of glass-framed letters. There, grateful parents had written gushing anecdotes about the restoration of their children's health thanks to Doctor Bennet and his pediatric gastroenterological know-how. "Do *you* ever vomit your food?" he repeated.

At least the door was closed, and of course Eden, bouncing slightly on my lap, couldn't understand. The only answer I could think of was "No." Or, "No, I don't vomit my food." I worried that if I repeated the word *vomit* as in "No, I don't vomit my food," he might think I was mocking him. Yet I couldn't think of another, better word, a word that would import that I would be the last person to vomit even if I was at the greatest vomit party ever and everyone one else was vomiting jubilantly.

Does he think Eden and I are bulimic? I wondered. *Munchausen syndrome?* I couldn't fathom his reasoning.

But a few minutes later I willed myself to forget that Doctor Bennet had asked me such an inexplicable question because he told me very definitively that Eden did have an allergy and yes, it was to dairy. That was it! After months of the pediatrician's belief otherwise, Doctor Bennet asserted, "Your son can't tolerate the dairy that's in his formula, and it causes him to reflux it." *Vomit, you mean.* It was that simple.

I wanted to cheer and, ironically, puke all at once. Puke up my stupidity. I was too happy for an answer and too furious at myself, an unstable combination of emotions. I felt so grateful to Doctor Bennet, and, later, other specialists, when they offered a reasonable diagnosis for Eden's unreasonable symptoms that I tried to not have too many opinions or questions about Eden's treatments. I didn't want to disturb these precious relationships by raising a green or red flag.

I ponged and then again pinged. I left my first pediatrician. The second pediatrician had a voice like a bell, clear and resonating. Admittedly, she had only an average knowledge of allergies, but she seemed empathetic, acknowledging Eden as a child with a food allergy. (As opposed to my first pediatrician, who later told me it was "very interesting" that Eden vomited far less with hypoallergenic formula. She said it like, "That new bookstore finally opened? That's *very interesting.* I might just stop by.") Besides, Doctor Bennet had told us that he would take care of Eden's allergy.

Even as we optimistically began our journey to safety with Doctor Bennet, Eden started having strangely opposing symptoms: His weight was still low but steady. Eden vomited far less often, though more than I would have liked, but his eczema worsened. His skin was so itchy that he rubbed his wrists on his high-chair tray and the arms of his stroller until the plastic was streaked with translucent red. Yet despite the bloody baby apparatus, in early December, Doctor Bennet recommended that I "introduce" milk back into Eden's diet.

Had I been feeling comedic (I wasn't), I might have deflected my shock at Doctor Bennet's pronouncement with the quick riff "Helloooo, milk!" Again, I wasn't, so I didn't. Plus I assumed Eden wouldn't be touching the white stuff for years. But Doctor Bennet recited statistics. To a parent already fatigued by her symptomatic child, a statistical citation was the medical equivalent of a hot foaming cappuccino. Doctor Bennet explained the high statistical probability of a child outgrowing the most common of all food allergies—dairy—within a year. At the time, doctors agreed that if not by a year, the vast majority of milk-allergic children outgrow their allergy by age three. However, the studies Doctor Bennet may have been referring to relied on milk-allergic children within a general population and included different types of milk allergies.

Between 1997 and 2002 (the year Eden was born) the number of children with life-threatening peanut allergies appears to have doubled.[4] The percentage of children with atopic dermatitis increased from 3 percent in the 1960s to 10 percent in the 1990s.[5] Asthma rates in children under age five increased more than 160 percent from 1980 to 1994.[6] In 2007 a study at the Johns Hopkins University School of Medicine found that children like Eden aren't likely to outgrow their allergies by elementary school, if then.[7] Moreover, in 2011 an article in *Bloomberg BusinessWeek* magazine would describe studies that conclude that children with moderate to severe eczema are less likely to outgrow a milk or egg allergy than are children with mild or no eczema.[8] And in June 2011 the American Academy of Pediatrics published a report estimating that 1 in 12 children in the United States have food allergies; the finding suggested that the severity of those food allergies was greater than previously reported. Those statistics mirror our experiences, and those statistics still feed my irrational regret. I have to wonder now, after the fact, how all those parents felt during the polio epidemic, when the first wave of children fell victim to paralysis. Did those mothers look back at their children's first signs of fever and wonder if they could have done something? Of course they did.

But Doctor Bennet offered precise instructions involving a progression from cheese to yogurt to liquid. There was no fine print stating that our actions, taken willingly, would lead to one allergic reaction and then others, a rolling landslide that would cause Eden to have anaphylaxis and that sickening rush to the emergency room within a month's time.

The funny thing about a diagnosis is that you can forget it isn't supposed to be an answer. A treatment can answer the question of how someone may live or die. According to *Merriam-Webster's Collegiate Dictionary*, the definition of *diagnosis* is "the art or act of identifying a disease from its signs and symptoms." That's all. After we slowly reintroduced milk according to

Doctor Bennet's orders and then stopped again because of Eden's adverse reaction, Eden ricocheted out of the emergency room over to a pediatric allergist who then diagnosed him as allergic to a seemingly endless list of foods and environmental allergens. Anaphylactic.

Despite some relief at finding a doctor who provided a detailed diagnosis, I felt that Eden's first allergist had a less comprehensible approach to treatment. While brandishing an EpiPen and literature, he reassured us with phrases such as "Trust your gut" and "You are the experts, but keep informed." Though I'm sure he was trying to boost our spirits, it felt like he was playing both good cop and bad cop in the same white-coated costume. I wasn't ready to be an expert because I could hardly fathom what he was saying. How is it possible for a child to be allergic to dairy and soy and eggs and nuts and beans and shellfish *and* some fruits? How? How to live with that? Our allergist cautioned us to avoid Eden's allergens, but when I went home, I found smoke and mirrors within that simple directive.

Smoke: I met my effortlessly groomed friend Liz in the playground. She was smiling, her long blond hair pinned back perfectly. Her handsome one-year-old, equally casual, munched on his Gerber Wagon Wheels, a puffy apple cinnamon "cereal-like" snack. Dutifully, I read the package. Hmmm. "Natural flavors." What is a natural flavor, really? Whatever it is, it must have something to do with apple. I tasted a wheel, and it reminded me of Apple Jacks. Watching us, Eden held his hands out eagerly for this enticing nibble, and I figured Wagon Wheels were okay. But I really didn't know for sure.

Mirrors: Another day I played it safe and made a simple lunch of pasta for both my children. But as I stirred olive oil into the second bowl of penne, I thought I might have used the same spoon to butter Dayna's portion. But then there was another spoon like it lying in the sink. Hesitantly, I dumped the penne in the garbage anyway. Was that right?

The phone calls to the allergist felt more embarrassing than my ambiguous decisions. The calls made me feel oddly guilty, like picking a dollar off the floor when no one is in sight. Wedged between the hamper and the window with the bedroom door closed, I began, "Hello. Thank you for returning my call again." Thank you. Always thank you. The appeasement. Sorry to bother you. Sorry for my seeming incompetence. I was always thankful, always sorry.

"As I told the nurse, it's just a food question. Umm, actually it's about soy lecithin. Oh? Lessithin? It's a soft *c*? I didn't know that, umm, as you could probably tell. Anyway, so I'm sure you would know this, but it, umm, lecithin seems to be in every kind of bread. Could that be a problem for Eden? He's been eating a lot of toast. Right now his skin is really bumpy on his cheeks and mouth."

Instead of words, it seemed I was only making sounds, my questions popping in tiny bursts of stupidity. "Oh, and umm, also, I have another question after that one. Eden, umm, threw up. Well, no, a spit-up? But, uhh, anyway, it was steamed flounder just five minutes into eating it. Remember how you said white-fleshed fish, but maybe not salmon, should be okay? Well, I wasn't sure, but he could have just gagged. It was so quick."

Eden's first allergist would begin, "What you're describing *should* be okay . . ." At some point he would have said, "However, there are unusual circumstances," and he always concluded with the affirmation "I truly believe you parents know best."

Later, I would try to interpret the phone calls with Drew. "He said tomatoes don't test that reliably on the skin. So ketchup . . . well, you could try it." Drew and I could spend hours dissecting the language.

Why all the analysis? I wasn't ready to be an expert. For one thing, while I was offering fewer and fewer kinds of foods, Eden still looked like he was having allergic reactions all the time. If I gave him a new kind of dairy-, soy-, and egg-free frozen waffle for breakfast, by three o'clock in the afternoon he was scratching at bumps on his forearms. But was he scratching because he'd had a bath just before and the water dried his overly sensitive skin? And why was he choking on my steamed-until-they-melt carrots if he was negative for carrots? Or was the waffle from before the potentially irritating bathwater also causing his stomach upset? Why he was vomiting up his food on occasion after an allergy-friendly meal? No one, not even our allergist, was telling us that we should be incredibly confused and that we really needed lots of help configuring a diet that would bring Eden to a baseline of health. We didn't know how Eden's "healthy" body was supposed to look or behave, so we didn't have a standard by which to judge his symptoms. Instead, our allergist was doing his best to empower us, and we just weren't ready to take charge.

My father spread word of our worries to the New Hampshire side of my family. I didn't mind, because I adore my New Hampshire cousins. We grew up sharing our beloved Brooklyn *bubbe*—the Yiddish word for "grandmother"—plus a few holidays and a seven-hour drive lying in sleeping bags and whispering in the back of a station wagon. Within a day, my cousin Lisa called. Lisa lives north of Nashua, surrounded by trees and hills. She turns her lights out during the day and pickles vegetables that she grows in a communal garden. Just hearing her voice made me crave her refreshing combination of New England–bred common sense, Jewish bluntness, and wholesome "give some back" living.

After she listened to my tales of Eden's merry-go-round symptoms, her spiritual advice was the same as that of my allergist: "Trust your instincts. Your gut will tell you what's right."

But there were things I couldn't say to a woman who had owned her own toolbox since she was seventeen. As much as I wanted to, I didn't tell Lisa that I'd somehow lost my gut along with my sunglasses and the last, lovingly penned birthday card from Drew. My gut was taking an ill-timed leave of absence. Instead, I hung up the phone and continued adrift, searching for a savior. I didn't understand then that all I needed was a doctor who knew enough to teach us that there were no magic answers, who had worked with enough parents like us to know what was needed, what was helpful, a confident guide as we learned how to care for Eden as best we could.

As I continued to clickity-clack away at the keyboard, Googling key combination words such as *garlic powder* and *welt*, friends told friends about Eden. One of them called me about a licensed nutritionist named Nancy Goldman. Though she practiced in another state, her website looked promising with its naturopathic approach to regaining digestive health. She had years of experience with children who had behavioral and cognitive challenges related to food intolerances. Even though I didn't think Eden fit exactly into her categories, I scheduled a phone consultation, hopeful, as always, that she could provide us with the answers. Also, I failed to tell our allergist about this consultation, which I soon realized was a mistake.

Late one afternoon, I sequestered myself in my bedroom with the phone and a spiral notebook on my lap. I was always prepared, ready to listen, write, and be a good patient. After reviewing Eden's history, the nutritionist suggested that Eden had gluten intolerance and something else. I scribbled something like "Esiophelliosis???"

In fact, Nancy Goldman was introducing me to a growing but little-known disorder called eosinophilic esophagitis (EE).* According to the American Partnership for Eosinophilic Disorders, EE is an allergic inflammatory condition. People with EE commonly have other allergic diseases, such as rhinitis, asthma, and/or eczema. She guessed that Eden had EE and an overlooked gluten intolerance. Oh, and Eden probably had a yeast overgrowth. We needed to build him up nutritionally.

"But he tested negative for gluten and bread, and cereal doesn't have any effect on Eden. I don't think I have seen it make him hive or throw up or anything," I countered weakly. In truth, I kind of wanted to be wrong. If I was wrong, someone else could be right, and then I would know

---

*Eosinophilic esophagitis can be diagnosed only with a biopsy.

exactly what to do. Nancy Goldman sounded certain that I needed to reconfigure Eden's diet. She suggested that Eden needed a special formula called Ultracare from a company called Metagenics, because it was based on rice protein. Is it possible to sweat from the front of one's neck? My first thought was the inward plea of mothers heard around the world: but now what will I make my children for dinner? There was so much to do: purchase gluten-free foods from websites, buy a bread maker, and contact a pharmacist she uses (ask for John) for a custom-compounded preservative- and dye-free vitamin mix. And yes, I should still stay away from an odd dozen of Eden's allergic foods while also avoiding gluten.

Still scribbling, free hand pressed against the sharp knots forming above my navel, I licked my lips to moisten my dry mouth. Then I heard Drew curse as he entered. He had come home early to take both kids out during the call.

Drew's frustration snaked into the bedroom. "C'mon, Eden, it's okay, we can't go out now, we're home. No, Dayna, coats don't go on the floor, you know that. Eden, please, just stop. I have to get my coat off, it's okay, yes, we can have TV. Dee, does it look like I can put it on now? Put your coat in the basket. Okay, Eden. *Stop.*"

Through Drew's litany, I heard Nancy Goldman ask, "He's not allergic to sunflower seeds?"

I didn't know. "He tested as allergic to sesame seeds, so the allergist said no seeds."

"These doctors don't understand food families! A sunflower has no relationship to a sesame seed! I'm looking it up." Papers moved, and she huffed. "Just what I thought. The closest food to a sunflower plant would be endive. He's not allergic to endive, is he?

It took me a while to answer, but she waited. Again, I didn't know. Instead of admitting my ignorance, I agreed: "No, he is not." Did her other mothers give their babies endive? Over Eden's cries, I heard something bang and then roll, plastic bouncing on wood. A cup?

"I want you to make sunflower paste to spread on his rice bread. You should make it yourself. Use a blender or chopper . . ."

I did it all. I bought packages from a site called Miss Roben's, an online allergen-free grocery store. *Who is she? Does she have allergies?* I ordered rice bread mix, amaranth cereal, gluten-free crispies, and a bread maker. A day later John, the pharmacist, called to assure me the vitamins were mixed with stevia, not sugar. "Whew! Close one!" I guessed.

We could afford all of it. Our insurance did not reimburse us for any of these costs, and foods that address allergies can come at a significant price. For example, laws for prescription formulas vary from state to state. A Medical Foods Equity Act would establish a national standard for coverage, but as I write this, it is still under congressional review.

Drew can be a fiercely protective and loyal person. He once lent an old friend a sum of money knowing that it probably wouldn't be returned because "he would do it for me if I asked." His sentiments about money are objective and expansive. I tend to fret about costs, and Drew often reassures me that money can buy time, it can buy ease, and it can buy facets of life far more valuable to us than material goods. But of course, food is material, and Drew and I could afford some kinds of health-care costs that many parents cannot.

There are two important provisions in President Obama's health-care program that should positively affect people with food allergies: one, children cannot be denied insurance coverage for preexisting conditions, and two, insurance companies cannot require preauthorization for emergency care or charge extra for out-of-network hospitals. The first change implies that if a child already has severe food allergies or asthma, he or she cannot be denied health coverage. However, if parents already have health insurance predating March 22, 2010, that insurance isn't required to start covering the child's allergies. Parents will have to either sign on with a new insurer or look into an altered plan with their employer. The second reform, regarding preauthorization for emergency treatment, is equally crucial since life-threatening food allergy and asthmatic reactions can occur anywhere.

I pay homage to our money as we recount our many advantages in these disadvantageous situations: "At least we can afford the therapy!" Or "Thank God we were at the kind of hotel with a top-of-the-line doctor." But although we know that money can buy our health, we also know that we can't count on money alone.

The FedEx packages arrived at painfully slow, *Pong*-like speeds. As each food shipment came, I cut the boxes open with Drew's Swiss Army knife. All the cereals and snacks tasted the same. If I were color-blind, my mouth would have known they were brown. I made the sunflower paste in my mini–food processor and spread it on Eden's homemade bread. It tasted good. Slightly nutty. *Uh, no, not nutty.* The Ultracare formula seemed less appealing. Eden pulled away from the bottle with a pinched mouth, like a twelve-year-old tipping down the dregs of his father's beer. Nevertheless, for the next few days I coaxed bits of bread and sunflower paste and Ultracare into him because Ultracare supplied "fructooligosaccharides and maintained friendly intestinal flora." It even had olive oil and sea vegetable protein.

One morning a week later, I saw my glass kettle bubbling, so I put Eden on the couch, propped by cushions. I was hoping for forty-five seconds of relative contentment to pour that water over a tea bag, get Eden's blanket, find Dayna's pants, and get back to the kitchen. A plan. I noticed that Eden looked particularly sleepy, staring into a clear globe that lit and spun at the push of a button.

Enough time to make beds? Walking to Eden's crib, I reached in over the wrinkled bumpers with their rows of happy giraffes. Weird. There were pebbles all over Eden's sheet. Pebbles. Ignoring the wooden bars pushing against my ribs, I reached in and picked one up between two fingers. It was squared off and about a cubic centimeter in size. Looking down, I saw that some of the grayish-beige pebbles were crumbled into dust. *Did he go to the sandbox yesterday?* Time gathered around me, and then it separated—a momentary centrifuge. *No. Not the sandbox.*

Then I just knew. I knew where the pebbles had come from even before I picked up the nasty nugget of impossibility and sniffed hard. The smells of digestive juice mingled with the soured yeast of rice bread, and a sliver of roasted chicken bypassed my brain and raced through my adrenals. I pumped with self-loathing as I held the parched and unnatural contents of my child's stomach. Eden had thrown up in his sleep, and I hadn't heard him. Or he threw up in his sleep and was so resigned to his physical discomforts that he didn't even call for me. Eden threw up these pebbles and slept among them instead.

I screamed for Drew.

Of course Drew caught up swiftly. He was a ready father: ready to be angry or mournful, ready for his share. He slammed down the bar of the crib and ripped off the sheets, threatening, "We're calling that Nancy Goldman!" He stuffed the sheets into a laundry bag with his back to me, his words streaming over his shoulders: "I'm going down to the laundry room now. This can't wait. I want to know what's going on!"

I am man. Hear me roar.

Then the phone rang, and I remembered my tea. Eden started calling, "Mama." His face looked no different than it had a moment ago. There was no evidence of his nighttime distress. He held his pale arms up to me as he always did. *I'll bring his blanket and cube stacker into the kitchen; did I forget to get honey?* I was irritated about honey.

Drew, back from the laundry room, silently opened a window. I can't say exactly when, in the five minutes between the sheets and the damp, cold wind cutting through the stuffy apartment, our mundane life returned to its normal motions. Drew and I had been so worn by all the minicrises, minihorrors all, that we absorbed this next development into our momentum. Eden was preverbal and highly allergic when we engaged in gluten-free dietary experimentation, and now I understand that that was the wrong way to learn anything about his allergies. This was our lowest point in Eden's illness. Instead of coordinating Eden's medical care or looking for solutions that were based on the care provided by our current allergist, we had covertly turned to a nutritionist to save us. We had looked for a new medical perspective in our intense desire to make our son feel better, and in doing so we had failed him.

When she returned our call, Nancy Goldman responded calmly, because why shouldn't she be calm? "Well, he is *sensitive*, isn't he? Let's take him off the Ultracare for now and strengthen his body. We need to give this some time."

I chose to listen. With the thin padding of her words and an hour's time, I accepted things that I would not have accepted before. Maybe Eden lay in the dark, vomiting with his eyes shut, rolling into different positions. Maybe he gave up.

I gave the program two weeks. But two weeks was too long. As we learned later, Eden was in the early stages of malabsorption, the "impaired absorption by the intestines of nutrients of food." He leaked foam and watery streaks into the diapers that he needed more and more often. I tracked his bowel movements for those weeks like a shit detective. By week's end the bowel notebook testified to Eden's quota of diapers—eight or more daily. It didn't make sense.

Now, of course, I understand. Eden may have had leaky gut syndrome. *Leaky gut* is the term some use to describe the altered permeability of the gut wall, which can be due to inflammation.* Those tiny holes allow larger food particles to leave the gut and enter the bloodstream. When that happens, the immune system interprets those larger food particles as new allergens. Or I wonder if his digestive system was as tired as we were.

---

*The term "leaky gut" is not a standard medical diagnosis. According to many alternative medicine practitioners, however, evidence is accumulating that it is a real condition that affects the walls of the intestines.

It wasn't until Drew and I took Eden to another and last allergist that we would learn that many of the recommended specialty foods we had fed Eden probably were "contaminated" with Eden's allergens. Though at that time there was no such descriptive labeling, there was a good possibility that those foods were crossed, touched, or contaminated by another food when they were made. Sesame seeds on a baking tray, almond particles on the bottom of a giant vat, or egg white stuck on a mixer could have contaminated any of the foods I was giving Eden, particularly since they came from small factories and processing plants. We learned that he was in fact allergic to sunflower seeds.

Soon, as Eden's diapers filled, he got hungrier. In one meal he ate three slices of rice bread and half a roast chicken down to the bones. Conversely, he wouldn't swallow liquids of any kind. Within a few days of his food in, food out frenzy, Drew and I called Eden's second pediatrician, Doctor Elliot, to confess our dealings with Nancy Goldman We couldn't face Eden's allergist with our unfaithfulness. Doctor Elliot told us, "I can't help with this" but to "hold on just hold on" and to "give him Pedialyte. . . . Is he still peeing, then we are okay if he is still peeing . . . he needs to be peeing . . . he really needs to be drinking more . . . try apricot nectar . . . he's still not peeing? I'll get you a referral to see a specialist. Now."

Another doctor. We pinged and we ponged. It was the last thing we wanted to do and the only thing we could do, the sum of anyone's emotions when he or she must, really must, see a doctor. And if we were going to bring our sick child to another doctor, well, we were going to do it right. Enough! We took charge in our own way. There was a shiny, dark-blue three-drawer file cabinet in the corner of our dining room. I used to keep my middle-school teaching lessons inside, neatly labeled "Coming of Age" or "Dialogue Prep." I had tabs with subcategories and folders for projector sheets. In fact, that file cabinet was just as I had left it when I stopped teaching after Dayna's birth. My hiatus from the classroom was supposed to end at some point after Eden was born, possibly even in his toddler years. But at that time, my concerns for Eden preempted any thoughts about my career.

Since the file cabinet was filled, the top was all Eden: piles of manila folders of medical records and tests; mailing envelopes stuffed with prescriptions; notebooks recording food, formula changes, and blood and urine tests; paper plates jammed between the layers of cardboard; and napkins with scribbles waiting to be transcribed. The stacks threatened to topple like Dayna's building blocks.

Envisioning our urgent appointments and Eden's inevitable ruckus in my arms as I met new doctors, I didn't know how I was going to review and pinpoint our concerns cohesively. So Drew and I took on Eden's health records, unwieldy as they were, and narrated a chronological health history. We began to gain control. For a day it was all we did. I'm sure at some point I helped Dayna tie her shoes, or wiped the counter, or bought paper towels. I'm sure.

We took down our files, records, and day calendars and lined them up next to the computer. We began "in utero" and painstakingly progressed through a cataloging of every formula, doctor, treatment, dietary regimen, and medicine. There was a weight and height chart in a text box, a numbered list of concerns, and bullet-pointed health goals. It was six double-spaced pages. We collated and stapled four copies, and I found a bright-red pocket folder to hold it all. Eden's story.

Did the story have a happy ending? Did Eden receive the most informed treatment available for a kid with his particularly virulent and severe allergies? The easy answer is yes. He was saved. We went to a second pediatric gastroenterologist at Mount Sinai Medical Center who, after examining Eden and taking his case, immediately referred us to an allergist in the Mount Sinai department of pediatric allergy and immunology. That department is home to the Mount Sinai School of Medicine Jaffe Food Allergy Institute and is one of the most esteemed allergy research hospitals in the country.

"I'm not convinced this is a GI issue," she told us. "I think his allergies are the real issue." How right that second GI was. The Mount Sinai Jaffe Food Allergy Institute is to allergies what Memorial Sloane-Kettering is to cancer treatment. It was where Eden needed to be.

After packing up slices of rice bread in Baggies (and later reading the hallway signs indicating that there was absolutely "No Food Allowed" . . . *Duh, it's the food allergy floor*) and after having our mandatory marital spat in the elevator and then compensating by playing the cheery parents ("Look, Eden, new toys!"), we were there.

Eden played with Matchbox cars in his signature style. Generally, he rummaged through toys quickly and used a single finger to touch one cautiously before moving on. He wasn't physically restless, just mentally. At fifteen months, he wasn't interested in walking. Concurrently, when he sat down near toys, he rarely attempted to organize them into piles or scrutinize particular features, as Dayna had done. So while he picked up those little cars and haphazardly discarded them, I checked out the other families and their children. There was a mother clad in a sari, holding a baby wrapped in a finely crocheted blanket. There was a slight little boy wearing corduroy overalls, pulling at a Peg-Board. Drew whispered, "You never see any fat allergic kids, do you? They are all so thin."

"I think you're right," I agreed. "Yeah. They must all be." Did that signify? We were looking for clues. Would this be the last doctor, the one, or just one more doctor?

It was a long, long wait, and we ran out of predictions before we met Doctor Anderson. Then she was all soft lines, with a rounded face and an even rounder, pregnant belly. Her *s*'s were elongated, and her movements punctuated with half nods. While she delicately examined Eden, we learned he needed a fresh set of skin and blood tests to determine his current allergic status. Were there any foods we were particularly concerned about? Hmm? You can tell me. Her soothing demeanor was miles away from our anxiety.

"He seems to be allergic to everything," we told her, hating how crazy we sounded. But the confession nudged us all closer.

"Well," she said, and smiled at us. "It certainly can seem that way. Why don't we wait for the test results?"

After some debate, we requested tests for avocados, peaches, and sunflower in addition to Eden's previously diagnosed allergens. We asked for sunflower because we suspected it might have been one cause for Eden's latest bout of gastrointestinal distress. Testing for sunflower seed was a problem because an extract for sunflower wasn't readily available. Apparently, no other parents had made their own sunflower paste as a curative for their allergic children. So Doctor Anderson disappeared for a few minutes, and when she returned, she reported, "They have fresh sunflower seeds we can use for skin testing." I wondered *who* they were, those test makers, those elfin creatures in a lab somewhere brewing droplets of walnut and scallop extract on miniature Bunsen burners.

The nurse held Eden's arm, cleaned it, and then wrote numbers along both his forearms. She applied clear drops of liquid, each containing extracts of different foods, including one with a visible particle of sunflower seed. Then she scratched each with a small needle. Sunflower was number "5." Eden's skin swelled up into familiar bumps, which, in conjunction with his blood tests, was the basis for a revised list of allergic foods. No fish, mustard seeds, or avocados but a green flag for gluten. Go gluten. However, the infamous sunflower, distant relation to endive, friend to all salads, was banned.

"But it is all much simpler than you think," Doctor Anderson assured us. She reviewed the intricacies of cross-contamination and articulated why indeed it was too soon for us to be experts on a child as sensitive as Eden. Doctor Anderson used phrases such as "what we have seen in our other children here . . ." Once she began a remark by saying: "It disturbs me that . . ." What I liked about her was that she *looked* disturbed. It showed me more than her compassion. It showed me that she would hold herself accountable for Eden's health.

With Doctor Anderson, we analyzed cooking and cleaning routines and the dangers of inaccurate labels and small-scale food manufacturers with nonstandardized cleaning methods. Flipping through our history, Doctor Anderson instructed me to be wary of the ingredient lists printed on food packages. Instead, I should call the companies and check their methods with a customer service representative. Conveyor belts and other machinery can have food residues and particulates. There was so much we didn't know. For example, did I know that one of the brands of canned tuna contains hidden milk from the processing sequence in which the fish is bathed to ensure a moist meaty texture?* No, I did not. Did I know that the brand of organic baby food I had used often was made on "mixed lines"? No, I did not. The significant difference between our first allergist and Doctor Anderson was vigilance and certainty. Doctor Anderson prescribed a hyperawareness regarding food avoidance, and when there was any doubt, she referred to herself as the authority, not me. Not every parent would welcome her approach, but for us and for Eden it was just right.

Eden was making loud and bored chucking noises out of the back of his throat. Drew volunteered to take him back to the waiting room, and I suspected he needed to escape so that his brain could spin the *shoulds* around—what we should do, should not do, should have done. After Drew left, Doctor Anderson continued with those *shoulds*—I should continue to bake my own bread because most store-bought breads are run through machinery with milk, eggs, and seeds. I should consult with the on-staff nutritionist, who would soon be known as the juice-box and first-run-cereal expert. I should wait at least a week between introductions of new foods into Eden's diet. As an anti-cross-contamination home appliance, I should run our dishwasher with abandon.

---

*This is no longer the case.

We left with checklists in our hands, forms to keep in an emergency and for teachers and babysitters, written instructions that were clear and precise. And my gut was finally telling me something loud and clear: for the next few years, I wouldn't be straying far from Eden's daily routines. Finally I understood. Eden had a condition that I needed to control as best as I could. I didn't have to reconstruct my life, but I wanted to. Also, I didn't have to feel stupid. Of course I didn't know how to control Eden's allergies. Even with Doctor Anderson's help, I would make mistakes. She wasn't a deity, but she was a better partner for all of us.

It was around that time that Dayna began using the word *properly*. I never figured out who taught it to her. When her various creations showed early signs of mediocrity, she would rip the drawings into shreds, knock over her LEGO towers, and emphatically pronounce, "I'm not doing it *properly*." And she would abandon the project. Though he was confusing and his condition was frustrating, Eden was a child, not a LEGO tower. When a child needs fixing, most parents don't walk away from the mess in a huff as much as we might want everything done properly. In our case, we ponged helplessly between doctors in our desire to fix Eden. But Doctor Anderson helped me trust myself again. And after I had worked with her for a few months, my gut told me it wouldn't be wrong to consider a new and third pediatrician, one who could support all of us the way Doctor Anderson did. My gut told me that my second pediatrician was getting lost in an increasingly busy practice and that Eden was receiving cursory treatment by her new partners.

Doctor Martin was famed in certain parent circles. He had a reputation for being "different" and "offering choices." Before Doctor Anderson, I hadn't considered him because (a) obviously I was tired of changing doctors, (b) he didn't take insurance, and (c) I was suspicious of his reputation. Possibly, he was too unconventional to keep Eden safe. Was he a quack? But then my gut reached back and gave me an inward kick in the pants. I could meet him at least.

Except Doctor Martin wasn't taking new patients. His Irish nurse, Maureen, has a warm voice, so two minutes after I hung up, I called back. "My son has severe allergies. They made him very sick. We see a specialist at Mount Sinai, but he needs special consideration. He really has been very sick," I repeated. I didn't even mention a daughter during my staccato plea.

Maureen responded in an angelic brogue, "Oh. Of course, then, I'll tell Doctor Martin about him, you know. He is interested in special cases, you know. Oh, yes. Let me call you back."

She did. Quickly. "He doesn't have availability for two months. November. But he wants to see you. He likes to help in special cases, you see." *Do I like him for that?* I gathered the tomes, mailed Eden's health history, and recorded our appointment.

One evening two months later, I was stacking plates into the dishwasher when the phone rang. I rushed to pick it up, assuming it was Drew calling from work.

"May I please speak with Susan or Andrew?" The voice on the other end was telemarketer-friendly.

I started to muster my cold yet firm telemarketer tone when the voice continued: "This is Ben Martin. I'm just calling to let you know how much I'm looking forward to meeting you and your remarkable son, Eden." Remarkable? I was too stymied to reply. *He can't make it? He's calling to reschedule?* He continued: "I just finished reading your thorough history and can't wait to discuss Eden's many complexities and to further your thoughtful efforts."

The kitchen clock read seven-twenty in the evening. Was he calling from his office or his home? Was this something he just did? Was it a thing for everyone? Even if it wasn't just for me, what a thing! My prancing brain returned in time for his next question. "Will Andrew be joining us tomorrow?" he asked, as if I had been invited to a tea party to celebrate my son and we would do nothing but nibble small, delicately frosted white cakes.

"Well, no, sometimes he comes to Eden's appointments, but he has work . . ." I wasn't sure if Drew's presence was expected. Suddenly I wanted to rise to whatever this occasion would be.

"Of course. I hope Maureen explained your first visit would be about two hours or so. Good. Do you have any questions for me? No? Fine, then enjoy your evening." And he was gone. Inexplicably, I wanted him to come back. I jigged my way back to the dishwasher and jigged through the rest of the evening.

The next morning I carried Eden down the brownstone steps leading into Doctor Martin's ground-floor office. Maureen pointed us into a waiting room. Well, no one else was waiting. There was a fish tank, a wooden boat, stuffed jungle animals, and wooden pull toys. Eden, at almost two, deserted me with his waffle blanket still on my lap and made his way to the giant wooden rowboat in record time. It was peaceful with his crawling and climbing, the gurgle of the tank filter, and quiet voices behind the closed door of the third room.

Within a minute, a mother carrying a small tow-headed infant came out. Behind her, Doctor Martin was dressed in white denim jeans and a black cotton turtleneck, socks and Teva sandals on his feet. His sandy brown hair waved just above his chin level. He smiled, and his eyes and tawny skin glowed with pleasure. Later I would learn that despite his youthful appearance, Doctor Martin was several years older than I.

"You're Susan! This is Eden! Welcome! I'm Ben." Then he opened his arms and embraced me. Now, I'm not a hugger per se. His gesture could have easily felt hippielike or simultaneously creepy and needy. But it didn't. He just appeared happy. And it seemed like a nice way to begin something that I had never realized was in fact a personal moment—the introduction of a parent to her child's pediatrician.

It turned out the toy room wasn't technically the waiting room (Ben didn't believe in keeping his patients waiting), so we just stayed there. Eden bumbled about, surprisingly content. Ben asked me some of the usual and some not so usual questions, and at first it felt like a bottomless effort. "What is Eden eating?" Ben asked. Oh, God. I had analyzed Eden's diet so many times. Somehow I had this conversation with neighbors in the elevator, with people in the checkout line at our supermarket, with untired people on the Second Avenue bus.

Inhaling, I began: "Lots of meat, some vegetables, some fruit, the ones he can have. Umm, no citrus yet or berries and stone fruits, that's a problem . . . my bread, crackers, umm, I found this kind that's like a Triscuit but not, rice milk, but not really much, so I worry about his calcium a lot, and what else?"

"Does he eat a lot of meat?"

"Yeah, he does, especially hamburger. I try to buy organic or kosher." Already I was growing weary of the sound of my voice, exhausted by my boringness.

Ben wrote as he answered. "That's so wonderful. I'm sure you are feeding him beautifully. Now, organic, even kosher, are of course great choices, but if Eden eats that much beef, he may benefit from the CLA (conjugated linoleic acid) fatty acids found only in the grass-fed beef variety. Those fats can help Eden regain some balance on inflammation and provide a host of positives. There is a place you can order from and read more, if you're interested."

"If you're interested." Ben's last words mattered more to me than CLA fatty acids or what salad mix those cows ate. *Know what? I am interested. Thanks for asking.*

Then we discussed the function of fatty acids and studies conducted on pediatric populations. This appointment took place in November 2004, two years before Michael Pollan's seminal book *The Omnivore's Dilemma* became every food-conscious American's compass pointing toward grass-fed and organic farming. Ben brush-stroked his thoughts, speaking like a peer, breaking information into useful and satisfying bites. In addition to Eden's general health, we discussed alternative therapies, the detriments of excess chlorine in bathwater, Broken Cell Wall Chlorella supplements, and parenting books. All options.

At the end, after we hugged once more, Ben handed me seven pages of notes written on thick, off-white stationery. The writing was scrawled but legible, and the pages were filled front to back with every iota of information we had discussed. Essentially, he handed me the visit, implying this was my time and my work too.

On the bus, I read the first page. It began:

Eden: 1) Wonderful 2) Allergic phenomenon—there are two therapies that purport to address the tendency for severe allergies . . .

Leaning back in the seat, I gripped the notes and pulled Eden closer. There are no saviors. It's up to us to find the right doctors, the ones who can help us save ourselves, and for the duration of my bus ride across Central Park the world held that promise.

Chapter 2

A TABLE FOR FOUR

DREW AND I MET YEARS BEFORE WE married and had our children. Though we quickly felt certain that we would spend our lives together, we had a lot to do first. Somewhere in our early time together there should have been a short gem of a self-help book titled *Twenty Things* Not *to Do in Your Twenties*. The tips would have included Don't Sell Your Car to Someone Who Promises to Pay You Later, Don't Accept a Job at a Top New York Law Firm a Month before Deciding You Don't Want to Be a Lawyer, Don't Drink Sambuca at Your Fathers' Second and Third Weddings, Don't Teach in a School Where Large Roaches Crawl the Walls, Don't Eat Pulled Barbecue the Day after Your Wisdom Teeth Are Removed, Don't Carpool with Fellow Graduate Students Who Won't Explain Why Their Licenses Were Revoked, Don't Think That Your Boss Is Just Being Extra Nice to You, and Don't Become a Vegetarian if You're Already Slightly Anemic. With so much collective life experience under our belts, we considered ourselves a seasoned couple by the time we became engaged, realistic about life's challenges and ready for the ride ahead.

After our wedding, Drew and I flew to Ireland to begin our married life in a world-famous castle-turned-hotel. If pressed, I could boil our honeymoon down to the scary bed and the brave sheep. Our ornate suite was a wedding present from Drew's family, and it was unsurprisingly majestic. But our bed! We spooned in one corner of a bed so enormous that I felt Drew was my only landmark in a vast and disquieting terrain. I had a frightening dream during our first night: the local village behemoth wanted his room back. I reached for Drew in the soft folds and found him.

After a few days we checked out of the castle, climbed into a rental car, and began a weeklong tour of the local towns. In contrast to our hysterical "we're too young to die" exchanges on the narrow roads, clusters of serene sheep dotted the countryside outside the car's windows. Remarkably, the sheep grazed on the surfaces of the steepest hills and nibbled contentedly even when perched nearly sideways at the misty tops.

"Why don't they fall?" we repeated with the conversational tolerance of newlyweds. "Whadaya think?"

We never bothered to answer our own question. Instead, we strolled the cobbled streets, pulled apart nougat-stuffed chocolate bars, made pub stops for hot sweet tea, and ignored the ever-falling drizzle. The obvious reason those sheep were so tenacious? Easy. Falling down wasn't an option. They had to eat. We all do. And our infinite hunger is all about the what and the how.

Neither of us imagined then that within a few years food and eating—of all things—would become such a challenge. Drew and I were fifteen months apart in age. We had lived together for five years and moved four times, twice to different states. We shared similar urban upbringings, extended and distended Manhattan family configurations. There were divorces and remarriages. Separately and then together, we had lived through old quarrels and buried anger: "No, she's not a half sister;

either someone is your sister or she isn't." "She gets Thanksgiving. He isn't invited." "They don't speak. He gets the second night." At that time in our relationship, if anyone had questioned our priorities, I might have raised my twentysomething eyebrows to the tune of "Uh-uh. I can think of some other things that are pretty important to us besides food!"

In time, Eden taught us not to overestimate our sense of control or underestimate the power of food. Though it had been low on our list of concerns before his arrival, food became our biggest challenge. We soon learned to respect the fact that food is a huge part of who we are from the moment we are born. We don't get to choose our family, and we don't get to choose whether our childhoods are marked by life-threatening allergies. Family and food are inseparable.

My parents were adventurous and enthusiastic eaters. My father's weekly cheese expeditions illustrate this: on Saturday mornings he always woke before the rest of us and drove swiftly across Central Park to Zabar's, the popular specialty food store, before the famed bagel rush. His punctuality paid off in the freedom to chat up the countermen or question the woman on the checkout line about their shared preference for extra-dark pumpernickel bread. My father enjoyed the hunt, whereas my mother's passions were best expressed in her own kitchen, surrounded by her vast collection of cookbooks. Decades before it was trendy, my mother kept a separate meat freezer in our prewar basement laundry room and filled it with cuts of meat from local farms. She would sooner whip up a soufflé than order in a pizza.

"So much!" my mother would say when she woke to the odd dozen wrapped white paper rectangles lying across the butcher-block counter. My father always bought too much cheese. "We can't possibly eat all that, can we?" Oh, but we would. Out came the thick dark coffee, fresh fruit, toasted sourdough rolls, olives, and sliced tomatoes to match each wedge. And when breakfast was over, my mother would carefully rewrap it and prepare her custom feta cheese marinade so it wouldn't dry up and crumble,

God forbid, like those tasteless supermarket brands. In our house, food was worthy of our time and effort.

In contrast, Drew's childhood diet was based largely on packaged foods: frozen vegetables, white bread, and the occasional Ring Ding. His cheese was orange, each slice individually wrapped. His mother cooked American standards such as pot roast and chicken breasts, but neither Drew nor his brother learned to prepare much of anything in their kitchen other than a toasted English muffin and a glass of Yoo-hoo.

Drew does have some warm and fuzzy food memories. His grandfather used to roast the Thanksgiving turkey to bring to Drew's parents' apartment. Since he would never consider taking a taxi, even when lugging a turkey sixty blocks uptown, the grandfather would put it in a box, put the box on a luggage wheeler, and haul the cooked bird onto the Third Avenue bus. Drew claims the trip uptown in the cardboard created a unique steaming effect. Every year, I've offered to re-create that je ne sais quoi flavor by sealing our turkey in a box for a few hours, but Drew never takes me up on it.

I emerged ahead of Drew but several steps behind my family in terms of gastronomic expertise. As a teenager, I duly served as my brother's second-in-command during the mixing of his signature German Sachertorte cake. But after entering adulthood I parted ways with my familial gourmands. After college, while my brother did a stint as a sous-chef, I avoided preparations with any of the following words: *brine, brown, reduce,* and *rub*. If I had to, well, I just cooked. The word *sieve* still sends me running. And when Drew and I began living together, we melded our tastes and backgrounds and found a comfortable middle ground.

The first time I stayed overnight in Drew's apartment in Washington, D.C., we forgot to eat dinner, and before we knew it, it was late. We didn't want to break our spell on the crowded streets of Adams Morgan. Instead, we walked from bedroom to kitchen holding hands, and Drew poured two bowls of cornflakes. The first spoon of milk tasted slightly sour, as if the carton had been in his fridge one day too many.

"Is it okay?" he asked solicitously.

"Great," I said, smiling.

"Hmm?" He grinned back, and we both finished our bowls anyway. We were in twenty-four-year-old lusty love. What did it matter?

Our early easiness was one of the hallmarks of our relationship, and it permeated our living and eating habits. During our first few years together, Drew was building his career, commuting to work long hours at America Online, and I was teaching while taking graduate courses. Home cooking just wasn't a priority given our time and budget. We met in the early 1990s, when a carbohydrate-heavy diet happened to be nutritional wisdom. "Sandwich night?" or "That salad?" we asked each other most evenings. When we tired of ethnic delivery, I intervened with simple bowls of pasta and jarred sauce, maybe with some bread on the side.

Then, in a two-year span, we moved back to New York City and had a baby. Once Dayna began to eat, she renewed a hunger at our table of three. Meals became far more interesting. As she became old enough to try adult fare, we fawned over her expressions as she tried the strange smokiness of bacon or licked at a smooth chocolate truffle. Suddenly, the grilled cheese at our local diner tasted novel. So *crispy*! An ice-cream cone was a sweet surrender to the sight of her rainbow sprinkles dripping onto the pavement. I was inspired to add meat to the pasta sauce and made the effort to mash potatoes.

Although food first reappeared on our family radar with the birth of our daughter, our fight with food began with Eden. First, there were those agonizing months when he did little else but vomit the contents of his bottle. Once Doctor Bennet diagnosed Eden as allergic to milk, we thought, albeit briefly, that we might be able to both manage his diet and enjoy feeding him as much as we had his sister. Within a few weeks of that diagnosis, he encouraged me to widen Eden's range of solid foods. His suggestion? "Some soft proteins. Actually, some of my younger patients like Eden take really well to gefilte fish. It's soft and salty."

Gefilte fish? It was odd and oddly tantalizing. Though it was an eccentric choice for a ten-month-old, it had all the right associations: dietary observance, warm religious ethnicity. God approved of gefilte fish! Ignited, I called Drew from my cell phone as soon as I left Doctor Bennet's. "I'm going to Park East right now. I bet they make their own."

Only a few blocks away, Park East is one of the largest kosher food stores on the Upper East Side. In Park East, the sound of rolling white butcher paper ripping and folding can barely be heard over the din of phones ringing and countermen yelling to each other, "Rabbi, what's the price on the brisket today?" (On the busy days, I had the impression anyone who answered them received spontaneous rabbinical accreditation.) It is kosher chaos. Regular customers gathered in random formations, waiting for their turn to place orders so plentiful that they could feed an entire team. Pounds of meat, gallons of sides, pyramids of boxes of the kosher Wacky Mac Macaroni & Cheese mix were shipped all over by parents who wanted their offspring to eat as well as their religious beliefs and wallets allowed.

At Park East, there are two kinds of gefilte fish. There is machine-made gefilte fish that swims inside a glass jar surrounded by icky, weird fish jelly, and there is fresh homemade gefilte fish that swims in a plastic container surrounded by icky, weird fish jelly. The fresh gefilte fish earned points for being incrementally less fishy and more fluffy, on the assumption that a lump of cold ground-up fish can be deemed fluffy. At Park East, fresh gefilte fish is the gold standard.

Our parents, who lived nearby, loved the gefilte fish thing. Doctor Bennet's suggestion had finally offered up some material for a fun grandchild anecdote. Eden hadn't given them much to laugh about until then. He was the third grandchild born into our combined family and the only one with questionable health.

"Honey, my friend Diane from California called yesterday, and I told her my grandson is eating Manhattan's best gefilte fish. Doctor's orders!" my mother recounted happily over the phone.

My father came over. "You got it fresh? The good stuff? He likes it?" He chuckled to himself. My father is a Brooklyn-born Yeshiva boy, but he doesn't accessorize himself as such. Sometimes it just comes out. He peered into our refrigerator for "just a smidgen" while asserting, "Eden knows what's good."

And Eden *did* like it. He smacked up his chilled fish and then fussed loudly when I picked him up from his high chair. I assumed he was hungry for more food, so with Doctor Bennet's approval, I moved on to the first-year basics: small bits of bread soaked in formula, cereal, fruits, and soft-cooked vegetables. Eden grabbed at it all, crumbs and moist bits of carrot falling onto his chin, while Dayna cast off attentive four-year-old glances, delicately twirling pasta onto her fork.

It was all "good stuff" until the memorable day Doctor Bennet suggested that I feed Eden some dairy in his incorrect optimism that Eden had outgrown that allergy. My notes from that appointment resembled an esoteric diet plan in which fruit can be consumed only an hour after meals and white wine is banned but red wine is unlimited. Anyway, I was supposed to feed Eden American cheese (or any processed cheese) for three days in a row. If he seemed fine, after the three days we would move to yogurt for another three days. The pièce de résistance? *Cow's* milk in Eden's bottle. It didn't look right even on paper, but I went with it. I wanted his allergy to be gone.

After a week Eden started to vomit the final yogurt serving profusely—opaque white liquid and solid drips off his tray and onto my lap. It was clear that the experiment had failed. But a stone was loosened from the dam; he vomited equally the next day too, and the next.

From then on, come mealtimes, in the few minutes it took us to squeeze Dayna's ketchup and eat a few forkfuls of anything, Eden usually erupted in belching gasps. Dayna watched as we jumped up from the white Formica table, pulling him wet and crying out of the chair while his thick aftershocks splattered onto our shoulders. We would disassemble the tray from his chair and carry it over to the garbage for scraping and pouring. We would wipe the chair, the floor, and the child. Then at last, after one of us grudgingly trudged down to the basement laundry room with the soiled clothes, the parent remaining might notice Dayna bent quietly over her plate. The sight of her bent there with nut-brown hair falling forward over her shoulders sent heaves of acidic love up my throat.

Eden had his first anaphylactic allergic reaction within a month of the milk experiment. Even now, when people ask me if we have ever had to use Eden's EpiPen or go to the ER, I may answer that it was terrifying or numbing. But those words are mere echoes of my silent scream that day, shadow sounds of Eden's body as it swelled helplessly.

In the numbing aftermath of anaphylaxis, Eden's first allergist asked us many questions at our first appointment. Drew and I answered a few of those questions proudly: "No dogs." "No wall-to-wall carpeting." "Smoke? *God, no.*"

But among the allergist's questions was this: "Do either of you have a history of allergies? Are any foods a problem for you?"

What we heard was this: "Did your son's problems come from you? Which one of you?"

My brief bout with food allergies were a distant memory. I woke up with a fat lip when I was eleven. Fat lips, actually, because both of them were big, swollen, and, from my vantage point, nearly vibrating. My mother took the morning off from work to take me directly to Doctor Shapiro's office, ten blocks down on Central Park West.

Doctor Shapiro was the only doctor I had ever known. Everything about her was sharp: her scent, her pointy face, and her jet-black hair. I imagined her bathing in rubbing alcohol, applying it behind her ears and dabbing it on her wrists between appointments. After determining that I was having an allergic reaction, Doctor Shapiro and my mother discussed the possibilities. Utterly relieved not to have to face my classmates with my giant fish lips, I swung my legs for the sheer pleasure of hearing the exam table paper crinkle underneath them.

"Have you eaten a lot of a particular food recently? Or anything unusual?" asked Doctor Shapiro.

"Honey, what about at friends' houses? You went to Jennifer's twice last week. Did you eat something different there?" My mother was a tad suspicious. She would know of any new foods in her kitchen.

Jennifer's parents were temple friends, but they were Sephardic Jews, born in Egypt and schooled in Switzerland. My mother was a Sephardic Jew with Turkish parents. *Big* difference. Sephardic women take particular pride in their native cuisine and culture. At Jennifer's last birthday party each child was given an individual mini Bunsen burner–like apparatus to melt cheese. They said it was a Swiss dish, one of their European traditions. Maddening stuff for my mother, who wasn't versed in their cookery.

"I just had some orange juice and a brownie when I was there," I assured my mother.

"Did you have a lot of brownies? Do you like chocolate?" pressed Doctor Shapiro.

"No. Well, yeah." Clearly, we weren't leaving before they figured out the cause of the allergic reaction and my swollen lips. And by the direction of the conversation, they weren't going to name last night's spinach salad as the culprit (the salad I loathed, the salad that begged for a pedestrian sprinkling of bits of bacon to save it from its stringent spinachness and that tart dressing my mother referred to as vinaigrette moo-tard).

"What about orange juice?" Then, turning her head to my mother, she asked, "Does she drink a lot of juice?"

That was when I remembered my recent after-school snacks. "Yes. Actually, I really like oranges."

My mother broke in immediately: "Are you the one who's been eating all those oranges, Susie?" My mother has always sounded shocked that there are things she doesn't already know. As an adult I have learned to make use of the phrase "this might surprise you" before telling her anything that might be vaguely shocking.

"Well, we have a box of them right now, and we don't eat dinner until late, so I have been eating maybe a few oranges a day," I confessed to Doctor Shapiro, avoiding my mother's eyes (about four oranges would have been more accurate). Inexplicably embarrassed, I sensed that we had found the answer.

Blame the southern migration of my great-aunt Ray from Brooklyn, who had sent her annual shipment of Florida navels. My mother, ever the lawyer, triumphantly confirmed her deduction when, within a few days of quitting the citrus habit, my lips returned to normal. I don't remember if I was told to take any medicine. I just didn't drink orange juice and generally avoided citrus for a few years afterward. I'm pretty sure I outgrew that allergy by the time I was in college, since I distinctly remember an evening splitting and devouring an entire pineapple with a boyfriend bearing one.

Drew, by comparison, had a more serious history of allergies. Plagued by severe pollen and mold allergic sinusitis since childhood, he sneezed his way through sleepaway camp and college. The change in temperature between a shower stall and a bathroom can bring seventeen consecutive sneezes, easy, out of his tautly wired shnoz. Various kinds of raw produce, such as apples and carrots, make Drew's throat and mouth itch. Almonds too. I used to doubt this eccentricity because he could eat apple pie unhindered, and I guessed he was avoiding healthy fare such as fresh fruit and granola bars.

Then one night, prechildren, we went to a vegan restaurant in the East 70s that was frequented by hip celebrities. The waitress recommended the Candle Café Cocktail, a combination of fresh-pressed apple, carrot, and ginger juice. After a few sips Drew began to squiggle his mouth around and back his jaw into his neck, not unlike a llama I once saw in a zoo. Then he abruptly excused himself to go to the bathroom to gargle. Distinctly unconcerned, I glanced about on the off chance of spotting Woody Harrelson or Demi Moore eating tofu piccata.

We didn't know it then, but Drew has oral allergy syndrome. That syndrome, which of course Eden had to have as well, is characterized by an itchy mouth and can progress to mild lip swelling. It's not life-threatening. This phenomenon occurs when someone is extremely sensitive to pollens. For example, Drew is allergic to birch pollen, and his immune system recognizes the protein cells in apples and carrots as similar enough to it. When those proteins go down his throat, his immune system literally goes for the jugular and instructs his body to release histamines, which in turn cause the itching. Sometimes, people with oral allergy syndrome can trick their immune response by cooking the fruits or vegetables, thus reconfiguring the protein (e.g., apple pie). Most significantly, unlike a true food allergy, oral allergy syndrome does not progress to anaphylaxis.

So between us, Drew and I have a few silly anecdotes and one stuffed nose plus an occasional itchy throat. We could consider the genetics of our parents, Eden's grandparents, as well. My mother has had allergic asthma since her twenties. As a result, we didn't have furry pets and she has spent her life on whatever asthma medications are available. Thankfully, asthma treatments have improved greatly over time, and Eden and my mother have been beneficiaries of that progress.

Sure, Drew's father and siblings have hay fever. But looking down our entire family tree, there aren't any foods or airborne substances that close air passages, cause bodily inflammation, and stop our breathing. So were our genetics to blame for Eden's condition? Maybe. Well, in part.

According to the Asthma and Allergy Foundation of America, if only one parent has allergies of any type, chances are 1 in 3 that each child will have an allergy. If both parents have allergies, it is much more likely—7 in 10—that their children will have allergies.[9] In contrast to Eden, Dayna would develop hay fever and oral allergies as she grew. But life-threatening food allergies seemed like a crappy genetic hot potato to chuck at your child.

After more months consulting with different specialists, late-night Internet sessions, and dietary trials and errors, we found our allergist, Doctor Anderson, who understood what to do for Eden. Drew and I were supposed to resume our former lives with the utmost culinary caution. For Eden, no dairy, soy, eggs, legumes, seeds, fish, nuts, peanuts, shellfish, avocado, garlic, or stone fruits such as plums. And for us? For Dayna?

Our meals became confounding. "Meal planning's getting tricky!" I giggled psychotically at anyone who asked. Tricky? Who was I kidding? We lived in New York City, for God's sake. There was food all around us, some of the best in the world. Everyone knows that living in Manhattan is supposed to bring the ultimate food freedom—you can satisfy almost any craving day or night. When I was in high school, instead of raiding each other's refrigerators after parties, we stopped off at all-night diners and food markets. In New York, it seems everywhere you look someone is eating something. Herds of teenagers roam the sidewalks while slurping down hot pizza slices, young women wearing business casual grip cones of frozen yogurt in one hand and their Gucci bags in the other, and toddlers are pacified when strolling with oversized deli bagels tucked in their chubby fists. On our square block alone there was a taco truck, a waffle truck, a nut vendor, two fruit stands, a halal kebab kiosk, and two restaurants.

All of a sudden I felt like everyone around me was stuffing his or her face. Suddenly it seemed truly bizarre that one of my closest friends was in fact a foodie. (Alison. Really. She trained in Paris, debones large carcasses with pleasure, and poaches apricots with vanilla bean when she's "kind of bored." Check. Check.) In our hubris, Drew and I hadn't thought of ourselves as particularly sophisticated diners, yet we had chewed our way through Omakase sushi tasting menus and eaten in many of New York's highly rated restaurants. Suddenly none of my previous labels mattered because through my new lens the world was filled with food capable of causing monstrous consequences.

In the months after Eden's Big Kahuna diagnosis of multiple life-threatening anaphylactic food allergies, we scrambled to keep track of his restrictions, scrutinize labels, and understand what exactly was to constitute Eden's food going forward.

Quite suddenly Eden turned two years of age, and that was exactly when Drew and I began to cheat on each other. But our transgressions were not with other lovers. As the extreme nature of Eden's dietary restrictions dawned on us, Drew began having hurried, fitful, one could say closeted relations with food. Open cartons of Chinese delivery, hastily refolded bags of corn chips—those were the lipstick stains on his collar. Most of Drew's lapses were inevitably unrewarding. If I didn't catch him in the act, I would find him clutching his stomach or bent slightly at the waist moments afterward. And I cheated right back. A quick dig down to the bottom of my stroller bag revealed dozens of crinkly dark chocolate wrappers and the broken bits of Bavarian-style hard pretzels. This was my preferred type of meal plan when my nerves outweighed genuine appetite.

Without intending to, I dropped a few pounds, which for me was bad. I've always been fairly thin and small. I don't get to chuckle or even nod when the woman who bends her fork into the ravaged remains of her child's discarded cake, her plastic prongs nimbly avoiding the clear red goo between the yellow layers, announces, "She already ate the calories! I'm just eating the rest." I can't come back with the expected, "But you're standing up, so it doesn't count! Like you need to worry anyway." I don't get to pat my hips and sigh. But Drew had always been fond of my size. The first time we hugged, he whispered, "See? We fit."

Drew isn't tall, but he isn't small. He has broad shoulders and a solid stance.

I felt myself drifting from Drew and all the meals we had taken for granted, and the divide widened. We had impure thoughts. We reminisced over past events: that steak we ordered at my brother's birthday . . . that salad we used to eat with the baguette . . . that place with those cheese biscuits. We eyed the Snickers bars on drugstore shelves like jewel thieves in a vault despite repeated vows to turn away from such distractions. Neighbors holding pizza boxes in the elevator were subjected to nasty stares.

Eden's diet wasn't our only dilemma. Explaining his allergies to anyone, let alone a young child, was another challenge. Most parents will agree that toddlers can fixate on that which is unattainable. For example, a particular ceiling fan begs to be touched, another child's bicycle bell sings out to be rung. Then there was food and our inability to articulate Eden's condition to him at the age of two. I didn't know how to elaborate the reasons the cereal boxes with round green stickers were safe but the ones with red stickers weren't. Eden will get sick from food. How sick? Die? We didn't know how to explain to Eden that though the three of us might want to enjoy black bean chili, lasagna, cold cuts, grilled salmon, maybe even a pizza delivery, his plate was to be limited for a while to, say, soft meats, vegetables, and home-baked bread.

"Dat! Haf *dat*." Eden would point at his sister's pancakes. But he couldn't "haf" it (or even touch it) because I still hadn't figured out how to design all his gastronomic substitutes to have a comparable taste or texture, let alone appearance. It felt cruel to eat in front of Eden; children's brains are like little machines, recording and calculating. Why program his memory for an experience that would be denied indefinitely? Plus, I wanted to help Dayna understand the importance of her brother's condition without giving her my fears or overly restricting her diet, a concern that would be validated within the year by Dayna's brief but worrisome self-restriction.

A cloud of shame hung over all my questions. Every time we brought Eden to someone else's home, I needed to inform our hosts that we would be toting his food or question them about food preparations. Although it was understood that I had to speak out, I struggled to get over my ingrained childhood etiquette rule: never ask what's being served. Though we were supposed to be constantly aware of food to keep Eden safe, both Drew and I had an uneasy sense that food just shouldn't matter this much. In any given situation we were always thinking about the food, planning the food, and discussing it with an intensity reserved for people who were *starving* or something.

Drew and I drifted into erratic, nearly erotic eating behaviors (think bread crusts dipped straight into the butter container and a few honey-roasted nuts tossed down our throats late at night before we tossed that "gift" in the garbage, rinsed our mouths, and washed our hands). Our stolen moments ruined any appetite we might have had left for family meals.

Like most couples that cheat, we didn't own up to it. Instead we pretended it was A-okay that our meals, along with a host of other family routines, were swiftly disintegrating. Some evenings we gave the children dinner first because neither of us could muster hunger. Sometimes, for a treat, we would take them out for some late fresh air. One of those nights we were walking by a bakery we had frequented for years, a quaint throwback to a time when our neighborhood was largely German-American. On the sidewalk, Danishes, buns, twisted cinnamon rolls, small heart-shaped cookies, and glossy black and white frosted cupcakes toasted our air. Of course, Dayna wanted a cookie.

I waited outside with Eden in our unspoken agreement to distract him from Dayna's indulgence. Drew pulled the glass door open while asking over his shoulder, "Do you want something?"

"No." I eyed the giant spool of string hanging from a metal fixture on the ceiling. "Are you *sure?*" he asked, both he and Dayna still trying to meet my eyes.

"Fine. A sample," I agreed, wishing he would just go in and get it over with. Samples were the broken edges and corners of that bakery's signature brownies. Those crunchy half-inch bits were deemed dispensable and piled onto a metal platter on the counter. The edges were misshapen, slightly burnt, chewier and crispier than the squares that made it to the display case. Much better that way, I thought.

Standing there in the cold, I fantasized about having samples like those to replace all my meals. Wide, open bowls with toasted bits lining the bottom, minuscule squares of quiche crust and roasted vegetables, maybe bite-sized lasagnas and Lilliputian portions of grilled steak. Cocktailish fare easily dismissed for conversation, a clear coral drink, or, in our case, a child's inquisitive gaze.

Drew returned with a bite of brownie and a Wiffle ball–size muffin. "I got you this too. It's late."

And Dayna asked with wonder, "Mommy, why did Daddy get you a muffin? Is that dinner?"

"Of course not, Dayna. A muffin would *never* be dinner." But it was. I ate at least half of it that night in hasty bits while putting the children to bed. Looking back to nights like that one, I've concluded that in marriage, eating often tells the same story as sex. A couple that goes it alone can't enjoy the feeling of mutual pleasure and is in fact in danger of becoming uninterested in each other's appetites. Drew and I had pared down our relationship to separate sustenance.

So many questions remained unanswered: Should I whisk Dayna off solo on weekly trips to the ice-cream store as was suggested in an article I read? Did I dare pull up to the counter for a soft serve with both children in tow? For how long will Eden think that graham crackers should be as coveted as M&M's? What would Eden eat on our weekly pizza night? Would the steaming smell of freshly baked pie be unbearable? Dayna's cute little playdate guests brought murderous uncertainties such as Goldfish cracker crumbs. Passover at my mother's was riddled with eggs, walnuts, and anxiety.

"We need to keep some of our routines for both children's sake," I urged Drew as weekends devolved into a rotating scurry of squirreled snacks and solitary meals eaten out of the range of young eyes.

"And anyway, other parents must tell the younger ones that the older kids eat different stuff, you know, 'big-kid food'? Like . . . uh . . . soda?" I trailed off, knowing that almost no one in my urban circle, including me, actually gave soda to his or her children. Obviously, our quandary was more complex, and so our discussions were inconclusive.

After some delay, we tried the clichéd marital salve—the much-acclaimed date night. It took us a while to contemplate leaving Eden for even two hours, but after much planning we took that step. After preparing Eden's entire meal, soup to nuts (well, no, not nuts), and reviewing the placement of his emergency medications, we would leave both children with our food allergy video–trained and experienced baby-sitter and walk briskly to restaurants. But no matter where we went, our attention returned to Eden. If my crab cakes arrived with a shiny finish, then, "We'll never be able to take him to France, will we? Butter is everywhere there." If Drew's chicken cutlet was pounded and breaded to perfection, we had to note the egg wash it had received before the crumbs. If, God forbid, there were children seated near us, we tasted nothing but our bitter whispers: "It must be nice to be able to treat your kids like that, huh?"

The EpiPen back home was the elephant in the dining room. It represented more than our fear for our child's life; it was a symbol for all that we could not experience as a family. On one date, I looked back on our months of nibbling, binging, and obsessing, and clarity struck me: we were trying to swallow our guilt, not our food. Our shame was stuck like a fish bone in our throats. Nothing could get past it.

We understood that Eden's allergies weren't our fault, but nonetheless, it felt like we had failed: we had made a child who could die from eating food—our food. It was such a poisonous emotion that we didn't know where to look—backward or forward. Backward was sorrow, and forward was the understanding that surely we would continue to screw up—to take unworthy risks or unnecessary precautions—despite all our efforts. We were starting a brand-new learning process but at Eden's expense. And now we all had to learn how to eat again. Sitting there, watching our waiter with a dessert menu, I considered a family antidote: could I find or make a food that tasted as good as our love?

The epiphany kicked in while Drew was traveling for work. A few days earlier, Eden had cleared a chocolate allergy prick test, meaning he could eat cocoa powder as long as it wasn't contaminated by his other allergens. It was an ironic success considering the rest of his forbidden foods. One night, after both children were asleep, I went back into the kitchen to bake. I was afire.

My first attempt resulted in a gummy and slightly salty "devil's food delight." I rolled three different oils around my mouth before determining that extra-refined coconut oil tasted richer, more buttery, than the recommended and ambiguous vegetable oil. I added an extra spoon of cocoa powder.

I hadn't baked many cakes in my life. A year or so before, when Nancy Goldman managed to convince us briefly that Eden was allergic to all things gluten, I had spent hours baking and tasting unappealing concoctions. For a few weeks later that winter, I had been the old lady who swallowed things: flies, stones, gluten-free tortillas—you know how the song ends. Although we all survived our blessedly brief Weissman gluten-free epoch, I became pretty insecure about my baking abilities.

This time, though, I knew the second cake was going to be the one (the cake that got the guy, the promotion, a few children, and looked fabulous doing it all) even before it came out of the oven. The clock on the microwave glowed 11:00 p.m., a digital spotlight as I leaned against the counter with my face hidden inside the bowl of batter remains. I once read a memoir by an author who loved to eat and cook but didn't particularly enjoy eating her own food. She wrote, "It was like having a conversation with myself." If that was true of me, as my tongue stretched to reach the streaks of batter stuck to the sides of the bowl, I was masturbating. When I went to bed that night, the rectangular pan was perched atop dish towels on our counter, tightly covered with tinfoil. Underneath the foil there was a four-inch square of empty space that flavored my dreams.

Drew was away for five more days. Every night I tweaked the recipe. On the third day I went to buy a better pan at Williams-Sonoma, and a clerk there tossed his head confidently, handed me a small bottle of powdered lemon peel, and assured me, "It will sharpen the taste of any batter." Every night I baked and licked the bowl and the next day shared the results with my stunned children. They could find no logic to this bounty.

But I knew what I was doing. I understood then that my childhood memories weren't merely punctuated by food. Although food mattered to my parents, it was also another way to show me that I mattered too. I can still taste the chocolate milk my mother brought in a half-gallon carton on picnics by the lake near our weekend house. Surrounded by weeping willows, she poured its sweet thickness into paper Dixie cups, and I tried to drink slowly, making it last forever while the arching branches rustled. My mother knew she had taken us to a beautiful place and made sure we wouldn't forget it.

Then there was the sparkling night when I was seven and my baby-sitter dropped me off at my father's office on Madison Avenue. He let me touch the heavy glass paperweights on his desk and then took me down in the double-door elevator, thirty floors down to Giambelli. It was an Italian restaurant made famous by its history of serving New York's mayors and cardinals and, once, Pope John II. Legend had it that Pope John ordered antipasto, risotto, and fish. I settled on a deep bowl of spaghetti and meatballs, Parmesan cheese scattered powdery and light across the velveteen tomato sauce. Every mouthful tasted like love. That was the same flavor I wanted my family to recognize when they ate my cake.

A week later, I greeted Drew at the door after his red-eye with a piece of cake and a cup of coffee. The early-morning sun pushed through our blinds, and his blazer still smelled like airplane upholstery as he bit into it. Too exhausted to elaborate, he could only say, "That is goddamn delicious."

I squeezed him. "I know. It really is. And we can all have it. And after a day, you'll see, the top gets gooey, kind of like a frosting."

All of us loved the cake. We unwrapped sticky rectangles from plastic wrap and ate it on park benches, melted and fudgelike from the sun. After dinners we ate it half frozen, a cake Popsicle, out of the freezer stash. We devoured it as soon as I could pull it out of the oven, crumbling with chocolate-scented steam. For the next few years, I brought it to every extended-family occasion. I made cake after cake, and we didn't tire of it. Instead we gleamed at each other and talked with our mouths full.

It worked. Eventually, that cake was a lasting step toward eating together as a family and eased the sting of the inevitable moments when we could not. The first time I took Eden to a birthday party and brought a piece of it, he asked me quietly, "Can I always bring this cake?" It was his inclusion in a world where he was different, and thus armed, he could forget about his differences as he jostled around the paper tablecloth with his preschool posse. I baked that first cake when he was about two and a half years old, and though he is seven as I write this, Eden still loves it.

Eden and the cake proved to us that food is not love. Love is admitting that eggless French toast "does feel kind of weird in your mouth, right?" and then heading into the kitchen to sit at the counter and make just toast. Love is finding an Italian restaurant where they never screw up Eden's food and going back again and again even when there are nights we'd rather eat anywhere else. Love is Dayna leaving the table wordlessly to wash her hands ("just in case, Mom") and returning to keep her brother company while he finishes. Love is the Weissman art of cereal mixology—

the ritual of combining our sugary and unsugary cold cereal into a happy compromise of taste and health and then rating and mentally logging the results.

In fact, once Drew and I started to look past our plates, love unabashedly revealed itself. Love is sitting across from three children under the age of ten in a diner when they volunteer to forgo their home fries for the sake of cousinly solidarity. Love is laughing so hard at the dinner table that water comes out of both children's noses, and it just has to end with "That's *enough!*" and giggled aftershocks.

Love comes out of my hands as I cook, reflexively reaching for fresh utensils, wiping down the counter, long after the children have left for school and I'm only making my own breakfast. My food safety habits are my love.

I think food is often mistaken as love simply because it can fill us. I proved to myself and to Drew that love can be nourished with food and then find its way to the table and beyond. But the family sitting around must feel cherished. They must believe they deserve to eat. Finally, we believed it.

Chapter 3

RESCUING BUTTERFLIES

Before we knew about Eden's allergies, we took a two-week August family vacation to Long Island. In our planning for the trip, all we knew was that the eight months since Eden's birth had felt embarrassingly hard, the kind of hard that made us secretly wonder if other parents would be better at taking care of a child like Eden. Drew proposed that we recharge ourselves outside the humid city, and we both wanted to make vacation memories for Dayna. At the playground sprinklers I caught glimpses of her four-year-old arms, which were slender and tanned in her T-back aqua-green bathing suit that summer; I wanted to pause long enough to drink in Dayna's arms that summer.

Drew fixed on a fabulous rental home filled with unfamiliar luxuries: tall white walls and ceiling fans, a spacious back deck, an oblong pool, an eat-in kitchen, and a Jacuzzi. It felt too big for the four of us, so a few months earlier we invited old friends to share it. Besides, our friends Rob, his wife, and their two children lived in Santa Fe, and we rarely saw them. I imagined Eden soothed by the quiet breezes while the older children built sand castles on the beach. Come evening, the adults would drink cocktails by the grill, our damp hair heavy on our necks.

At that time I was unknowingly feeding Eden a baby formula to which he was allergic ("it's just reflux"), and his digestive system was in chaos. I couldn't see inside him and didn't understand that his geographic locale was irrelevant. No matter where we took Eden, he couldn't feel better any more than Drew and I could do it better. After a two-hour drive along the Long Island Expressway we turned off and drove on smaller roads to the paved driveway of the house. For the remainder of our first day I did little else but jiggle-jog Eden up and down the wide wooden stairway and out onto the lawn so that he wouldn't cry and vomit on the plush Persian carpets. That first evening I laid Eden softly on our bed to change his diaper, anxious about the prospect of soiled thousand-thread-count sheets and Dayna's unpacked suitcase. *He'll feel better tomorrow.*

In the two weeks that followed, the sun broke the dawn's haze every day around eight o'clock. The ocean water rolled in and out just over a mile down the road, and the air was lush with salt. But Eden was not so peaceful. The fresh air engorged his eyes. He wouldn't nap anywhere except the backyard tree swing with its gently rhythmic sway. So there he slept while I leaned against the broad trunk, dozing beneath the branches. He woke crying, unrefreshed. Drew and I held Eden and rubbed his back most of the remaining waking hours of those bright days.

"What made you call him Eden?" Rob asked one morning as I stood dangerously positioned with my half-empty coffee mug in my hand and Eden in the crook of my elbow. At arm's length was one more unexpected perk of the perk-filled house: a wall-sized coffee machine called a Capresso. It had a stunning mechanism. At the push of one button it flowed with espresso and cappuccino. Push, drip, drink.

Eyeing Rob's fresh foam, I answered, "Well, we wanted an E name for my mother, and after 9/11 Drew sort of wanted a Hebrew name. Eden means 'delight' in Hebrew."

Just then Eden began making these chucking noises, angry little exhales through his open mouth and nose.

"But he's not really living up to his moniker these days, is he?" Drew interjected almost saucily. The heady combination of sea air and our legal liquid drug had momentarily restored my husband's humor.

"Nah, not really," Rob agreed, watching Eden's grunts escalate into cries as he pointed at the screen door for a predictable two-step in which I carried him outside for a twenty-second reprieve until, unappeased, he pointed to go back in.

"Ta-da! And we're back!" I mugged on our return.

"Seems more like a Murray to me. Like a tiny old man named Murray. C'mon, Murray!" Rob cajoled. "Cheer up, buddy! We really do love you!"

Rob's remark echoed a few months later, the month after Eden's first birthday and his trip to the emergency room. I began to wonder if in his short life Eden's health issues had traumatized him. Was he in some way acting like a grumpy old man because of his experiences with allergies? I noticed this: Eden dropped things—bottles or cups or little plastic toys, stuff most babies liked to hold. When I held him up under his arms, he wouldn't place his feet down flatly. Instead, he curled them upward so that I would hold him or just let him sit up. And at the slightest noises, nothing noises such as the recycling room door clicking shut outside our apartment, Eden would pivot his head rapidly and clutch my forearm with an iron grip. Other triggers that brought on his signature head swivel/grab of terror move included doorways and large and open settings such as playgrounds. How was I supposed to spot Dayna as she finessed hand over hand on the horizontal bars if her brother cried at the sight of those metal gates?

Why wasn't Eden crawling around and exploring the big living room world or, as Dayna used to, chirping those noises through the monitor as Drew and I listened rapturously? Where were Eden's babbles? Eden did hone in on one activity. He liked it when Drew and I draped him over a waffle-weave blanket on our shoulders. Then he would rub his cheeks on that particular fabric while we walked and walked. "Wheef, wheef," it sounded like as I paced the apartment. When Eden was especially itchy, it sounded like "Wheef, wheef, wheef, wheef!" As an alternative interest, Eden was very happy in his stroller, especially if it was numbingly cold outside. I circled and pushed, entangled in a sensation of fresh and unending devotion.

Thoughts and legs equally wobbly, I wanted to believe the consolations of my friends and family. My brother weighed in: "Sam isn't sleeping well either. I know it sucks. I'm so tired too." But his son, Sam, who was just a few months older than Eden, wore a perpetual smile and gummed any object that couldn't run away.

"Rose used to shriek herself to sleep every night at that age," revealed Emily, a fellow preschool parent and a mother of three. "It's normal."

"Max still won't go to birthday parties or fairs," confessed Anna, my former college roommate. "Clowns make him beyond psychotic."

Returning to the lobby from our stroller marathons, I entertained the wise reminders of neighbors as they offered up sage clichés: "Well, when I had my baby, I thought he/she would be sucking his/her thumb/carrying that bottle/carrying that piece of crap at his/her college graduation. But I was wrong."

Was I right to fear that Eden would defy popular wisdom, that we would be wheefing and walking him in a numbed state of mental inertia forever? Was something else amiss besides his terrible allergies? Eden had moments, whole days even, when he acted more or less like a . . . baby, when he stealthily transitioned from banging a pot on the kitchen floor to upturning a full box of Cheerios or bobbled his head in pride as we exclaimed over his "Big Boys" jeans with a whole five inches of inseam. I wanted to believe those moments were his reality, not his exception. As that second winter of Eden's life continued, Drew and I debated his mental development even as we were busily decoding the causes of his chronic and spontaneous allergic symptoms.

I knew this much: I knew that Eden had allergies, and Doctor Parks, our first allergist, had mentioned that Eden showed a high histamine level on his blood test results. Did I have any idea what that meant? Not really. During that period, I had morphed from Susan Weissman to She Who Does Not Want to Ask, and I couldn't absorb the smaller details at the rate I needed to during doctor visits.

I began to have a better understanding of histamines when we started seeing Eden's second allergist, Doctor Anderson. Eden was about eighteen months old, and I was able to concentrate on the specifics of his issues. I had begun reading the body of available medical literature on allergies. For example, Eden's total IgE (immunoglobulin E) levels were measured at the same time his annual allergy and blood and skin tests were done. IgE antibodies are produced in response to allergens. What's an allergen? Anything our bodies decide to fight rather than accept. An allergic reaction is activated by the immune system, which is designed to protect us from harm in the form of threats such as disease and parasites. Allergic conditions include asthma, allergic rhinitis (hay fever), food allergies, and atopic dermatitis (eczema). All these allergic conditions begin when our immune systems produce a protein called an IgE antibody in response to a foreign substance. The offending stuff could be pollen, food, or medication. Each IgE antibody has an antenna and radarlike ability to "see" its enemies. The IgE antibodies sit on another substance called mast cells. Mast cells are like naughty children that come out to play tricks during allergic reactions, and we have a lot of them in our skin, lungs, digestive tract, mouth, eyes, ears, and nose.

When the IgE antibodies, which are perched on top of their mast cells, see an enemy, such as proteins from a swallow of milk, many of them will come together to bind proteins and cause the mast cells to release histamines to attack the milk protein. The histamines and other chemicals dilate our blood vessels, which leads to fluid leaking into our skin tissues. That, in turn, irritates our nerve endings—causing swelling, itching, and pain—and creates heat.

When Eden had his first set of allergy skin-prick tests, the red bumps on his arm registered as a triple response. A triple response is evidence that chemicals have been released, which creates (1) a bull's-eye "red spot" as a result of vasodilation; (2) a "wheal," or a raised, itchy area of skin; and (3) a "flare" of diffused redness surrounding the bull's-eye.

Some people make lots of IgE antibodies the very first time they are exposed to a substance. Those antibodies indicate that people are "sensitized" to a particular food substance, but those individuals still may not exhibit the clinical symptoms of an allergy. That is why sometimes people have positive test results without having reactions with exposures. But if clinical symptoms are displayed, those IgE troublemakers will get better and better at recognizing and reacting against substances. IgE antibodies are like soldiers in training, and they can multiply and become more efficient with every significant exposure. Eden's allergy test results proved that there were growing armies waging wars in his small body.

One mild February day, Eden had just begun a nap in his crib and Dayna was on a playdate. I decided to organize a forgotten bookshelf. (Resting was and is not my strong suit.) I came across a book of word origins I had used when I was still teaching English. Silently reminiscing over my lively classroom—"Does anyone know the original meaning of the word *conflict*? It might offer a clue to this chapter of *The Outsiders*."—I thumbed open the table of contents, read "Archaic Medical Terms," and flipped to that section. I read a term called *rising of the lights*.

Historically, *rising of the lights* is synonymous with the croup, a modern word for an upper respiratory infection in young children. In the nineteenth century the croup was a common cause of death for children three and under. So *rising* referred to any inflammatory swelling, and *lights* was an older word for "lungs." So rising of the lights was also defined as "the morbid sensation of something moving from the periphery toward the brain."

I could almost hear the spastic coughs of those sick children. Did they feel their pain rising as they made one last attempt to pull air through swollen throats and clogged lungs? Was that the "morbid sensation" mounting from their foundering outposts of skin, organ, and blood toward their young brains?

A few feet away, on our refrigerator, I had fixed a standard medical form with a checklist titled "Authorization of Emergency Treatment." There was one column headed "Symptoms" and an adjacent corresponding column for "Medication." I was told to keep this form close to Eden at all times. The instructions on the top read as follows: "If you *suspect* that a food allergen has been ingested, immediately determine the symptoms and treat the reaction with the corresponding medication" [italics mine]. Here are a few examples:

Throat—Tightening of throat, hoarseness, hacking cough—
Antihistamine & Epinephrine
Gut—Nausea, abdominal cramps, vomiting , diarrhea—
Antihistamine

The last symptom in the symptom column read as follows:

General—Panic, sudden fatigue, chills, fear of impending
doom—Antihistamine

Fear of impending doom. It seemed to me fear of impending doom was indeed a morbid sensation. A kind of pain. But according to Eden's emergency treatment form, only antihistamine should be used to alleviate this impending doom. During any minor allergic reaction Eden may have felt impending doom and I may have given him Benadryl for a few visible hives. In other words, he might have felt impending doom and I wouldn't have known it.

I sank down on our tile kitchen floor to think. Doom isn't pain. Doom is danger. It's dread; it's the fear of what is coming—dread of the unknown.

Then I wondered how often Eden felt physical pain. Eczema often is described as painfully itchy. Do hives hurt? Certainly anaphylaxis must involve some level of pain. Did those croupy children just know that death was coming? And what about my Eden? Has he been trying to protect himself from everything—from pain and the subsequent doom? Twenty-five years ago a doctor at John Radcliffe Hospital demonstrated that when operations on newborns were performed under minimal or no anesthesia, it produced a "massive stress response," releasing a flood of fight-or-flight hormones such as adrenaline and cortisol. Potent anesthesia, he found, could reduce that reaction significantly. Doctors had assumed that newborns' nervous systems were too immature to sense pain. Yet newborns who received anesthesia during an operation had lower levels of stress hormones, more stable respiratory and blood sugar readings, and fewer postoperative complications. Anesthesia even made them more likely to survive.[10]

For weeks Drew and I had questioned Eden's behavior, questioned whether we wanted to wave one more red flag over our child. At that moment, contemplating Eden's potential for physical and psychic pain, the debate was over. I picked up the phone and called Doctor Elliot, his second pediatrician. And when the doctor called me back, she asked the right questions: "Is it that Eden *won't* let you put him down or you sense that he *can't* let you put him down? Is he controlling you or is he controlling his needs?"

To which I answered, "Both. I think. But I'm sure he *can't* be away from us and feel normal. He acts too afraid." Together we split the hairs of normality.

Doctor Elliot's conclusion was far from archaic. She told me she suspected that Eden had sensory issues. That was indeed a modern term, a term I'd heard but never needed to pay much attention to previously.

I learned fast. Some of the signs of sensory issues or sensory integration disorder (SID) are oversensitivity to touch and sounds; a tendency to be easily distracted; impulsivity, or difficulty in making transitions from one situation to another; inability to unwind or calm oneself; and delays in speech, language, or motor skills. One therapist described it as "the inability to process and make sense of all the information coming in through your five senses and to make an appropriate response."

Doctor Elliot told me about a service called Early Intervention, which is a New York State–funded social service that offers therapeutic interventions to children under age three. To qualify, early development evaluators observe children with their parents and ask questions about their health and behavior. On the basis of our conversation, Doctor Elliot believed that Eden would qualify for Early Intervention. She gave me the name and phone number of the agency.

After I hung up, relief arm-wrestled with new alarm that Eden couldn't (not *wouldn't*) negotiate his one-year-old world. I tried to quiet my mind with the idea of help. We will get him help. But how do you give therapy to children under the age of three? In momentary hysteria, I conjured an image of a toddler lying atop the proverbial Freudian couch, her shiny Mary Jane shoes dangling as she discussed her hidden objections to shape sorters and the emotional implications of sidewalk chalk.

And then, my bottom still planted on those tiles, the word *autism* appeared as if it had been waiting in the wings for a stage entrance into my head. But no. No. Eden wasn't autistic; even then, my confidence glaringly weak, I was sure. But the characteristics of autistic children and the symptoms of SID are easily associated. It was early 2004, and all around me parents, pediatric doctors, and the media were invoking autism and Asperger's with regularity. There are good reasons why SID and autism can seem alike: although children with autism don't always have a sensory integration disorder, many autistic children do show signs of an SID. But there is not a conclusive tendency toward autism in children who have SID. In other words, SID can exist without autism but autism often exists in conjunction with an SID.

Within a few days, I filled out the state-issued Early Intervention applications and requested copies of Eden's medical records. Doctor Elliot warned me that completing the New York Early Intervention application is a lengthy and careful process and suggested that (if I could afford it) I find a private occupational therapist during the expected interim. Her advice was welcome since I'd never dealt with a governmental agency before. I knew little about the inner workings of the process. I never went to the agency's office or met the administrators who were involved in processing my paperwork.

And so in the middle of that frantic season, a spring spent learning as much as we could about Eden's allergies, with Drew and I holding hands as we ran through gluten-free confusion in a panic that finally landed us at Mount Sinai Medical Center, I began calling around for private occupational therapists. We could afford a few private therapy sessions while the New York State approval process took place. I found a highly recommended occupational therapist named Marla.

I took Eden across Central Park to Marla's facility and waited with him in a narrow front room facing West 86th Street. I watched the cars stop and start and massaged my wrists, which were sore from midnight pacing with him in my arms. Eden cried when I sat him on the floor near the toys, and so I put a Fisher-Price garage on my lap for him to play with.

The plastic corners jutted into the flesh of my hips, and there were honking noises when I shifted.

The term *occupational therapy* has a wide variety of definitions, though generally it refers to assistance for the disabled or convalescing so that they can achieve or maintain their functional daily living at a level that allows as much independence as possible. Of course, at one year old, Eden wasn't supposed to function independently. For young children, occupational therapy boils down to a studied practice of play activities to accelerate delayed development in fine and gross motor skills.

Marla called us into her gym. Smiling, with dark hair, she acknowledged me briefly, and I took her lead. I melded my words into the background of her coaching. "Look, Eden. Look at this. At how much fun it will be. Just look at *that*." Marla focused on giving Eden a tour through oversized vinyl pillows and the various trampolines, swings, and balls. One of her swings looked like a hammock, and in a brief but overwhelming moment of fatigue I imagined myself napping in it.

In the first session Eden wouldn't put his feet down. He was a swinging monkey, scooping his legs up and under him and clutching my arms. Clearly, he wasn't the only child with a foot fetish because we stood on a wide range of tiling from textured bumps to swirls. *Floor* was a big deal at Marla's.

As Marla tried to engage Eden with her toys, he pointed mutely, indicating that she, not he, should throw the ball or push the button on Big Bird's head. *Go ahead. You do it. I'll just watch.* But Marla had his number. Before she did anything for Eden, she asked him, "Marla do first? Then Eden? Marla do? Then Eden?" In the sessions to follow, that would be her slogan: "Marla do?' Marla do? *Now* Eden do."

Back home, I boiled pots of rice, sliced bananas, poured Cheerios, rewrapped the string cheese Dayna left on her plate, bought more Aquaphor ointment, left a voice mail or two for Eden's doctors, washed the bottom of the rice pan again, and filled bathtubs. And once a week I took Eden to Marla, where they got equally busy.

There were moments when Eden surprised me by complying with Marla's persistent "Now Eden do?" Sometimes he seemed to enjoy thrashing about in her giant box of Styrofoam bubbles. Occasionally he wanted to kick bright balls and pull plastic levers. He didn't smile in response to Marla's sunny squint, but sometimes his face would brighten vaguely, as if the world looked like a place he might want to be.

Shortly after Eden began seeing Marla, I was called by the administrator coordinating Eden's overall care and learned that she had assigned him a social worker. Her name was Julie, and her job was to coordinate Eden's evaluation process and his therapists if he qualified for the program. The day Julie came, we sat at the dining room table and she stacked piles of papers and folders. While Drew and I passed sheets to each other, Julie explained that more evaluators would come to observe Eden. She explained Eden's legal privacy rights and our parental rights. Julie's glass of ice water sweated onto its clear coaster while I signed reams of paper and Drew held his hand out for my pen and blinked.

As promised, eventually evaluators followed Julie. And by the time the Early Intervention evaluators were ready to meet Eden, we had our current allergist, Doctor Anderson, to help us grasp the tumult in his body. The evaluators came to our home, sat on our soft mauve rug with their legs crossed, and asked us questions. Oddly, Eden rarely cried when they were there. Drew took time off work for those appointments, but even with him there, sometimes we struggled to find accurate answers. "When did Eden roll over—begin to form words—return facial expressions—point at objects?" the evaluators asked. Six months, no, five. Nine months. No. A year? Yet I could remember each of his allergic reactions with clarity.

"What does he do? What does he like?" Well. Drew and I had a firm grip on what *we* did. We told them about Marla, and we told them that when Eden cried, we held him, and when he jumped and stiffened at noises, *we* held him tighter. We told them that we had rewired our schedule around his persistent needs, carrying him to different windows in hopes of spotting an interesting pigeon or garbage truck. We told them that when my arms ached by early evening, Drew and I took turns pushing the stroller on the cold, dark streets. And sometimes on those walks I would try to take Eden into the supermarket to wander the warm aisles and read food labels, but he would usually cry because, like balloons and grass, stores made him cry. We told them all we knew.

The evaluators confirmed that Doctor Elliot and Marla were correct and that Eden was showing signs of sensory integration disorder.

They told us he might have other delays as well: "Definitely needs feeding therapy." More evaluations were needed.

"Uh-huh," we said together. "Uh-huh."

And then the evaluators promised us that therapists would call soon. We never saw the evaluators again. In the weeks of waiting for the therapists to call, I remember one morning when Dayna followed me from room to room, trying to keep my attention long enough to finish recounting her previous night's dream. Without pausing, she offered lengthy descriptions of losing dolls and rescuing butterflies. I don't remember if I listened that day or even asked a question. Other days I remember how I was too busy.

And then, just like that, Eden's first therapist called. "Hiiiyy! I'm calling about Adan Weissman!" a voice chuckled.

"Hi?"

The therapist's name was Laurie, and though she had my contact information, the social service agency hadn't sent her any of Eden's paperwork.

"So you need to stay on them," Laurie went on. "I can't start without paperwork, but let's set up some times anyway. Openings are so limited! And don't worry. If you stay on them, I'll get it at some point. Now, what are his main issues?"

I didn't know where to begin, where to find concrete moments in Eden's health saga, his allergic lifetime. "Well, he never liked to grasp or hold anything like toys or his bottle . . . umm, we're working on keeping his feet on the ground."

Laurie replied merrily, "Don't worry. I know your son. I'm working with a little boy just like him a few blocks away."

We fixed a start date.

After four or five phone calls to Julie the social worker, paperwork issues cleared. Laurie bounced into our foyer one afternoon, slinging a fuzzy fleece jacket over her shoulder. "Hi there. Hi there!" She greeted us sequentially. Eden looked up from his seated perch in front of our media hutch, where he was pulling out and tossing DVDs over his shoulder. That first session Eden and I sat side by side while he squeezed Laurie's squishy balls and pulled obligingly at her serrated plastic tubing.

During her second session, Laurie announced that we should have a brushing routine for Eden. Marla had explained brushing to me when she had tried it. Brushing is a common technique used for children who have a sensory integration disorder. Using a specific brush made from soft plastic, you make firm, brisk movements over most of the body, especially the arms, legs, hands, back, and soles of the feet, for three to five minutes six to eight times a day. The purpose of body brushing is to rebalance the tactile senses. Unfortunately, it made Eden's eczema itch and flair. So instead, every day I rubbed body lotions on his skin in a similar fashion.

"But it's not the same as brushing him at least six times a day," Laurie advised as she draped Eden headfirst over a balance ball, rolling him slowly back and forth. "He'll get used to it." She lowered his feet to the ground and held out one arm. "Start here and then do his legs, front and back. Don't do his face, though." She pulled Eden's sleeve up and stroked downward slowly.

Eden pulled his arm away, and she pulled it back confidently, lowering the brush. "You'll get used to this, buddy. Right? And Mommy is going to do it too!"

But I couldn't. Every time I began that process of brushing Eden's body, he started to cry. And after all Eden's body had been through, the repeated violations of foods and medicines, I could not muster the faith to believe that his cries were transitory responses. I felt like I was breaking the trust of mother to child, the trust of touch and skin. But Laurie's relationship with Eden was far less complicated. She brushed Eden weekly while he watched an Elmo video. Eden would sit atop a balance ball, "building his core strength," while Elmo jabbered at his fish tank and sang his "la, la, *la*, la" song.

Laurie was supposed to be joined by other therapists. Eden had been evaluated for feeding and physical therapy, and we were told he needed both. I was especially focused on his need for feeding therapy. Since his diet was restricted, it was stressful when he continued to gag up his meals. I imagined him losing crucial nutrients, reliving his allergic reactions.

After a few more weeks of waiting, I called Julie. She said something surprising: "Actually, I'm leaving this position to train to become an occupational therapist too." Of course I thought that was wonderful except . . . what about Eden? And after Julie left, Eden's case seemed to get sucked into a vortex of disappearing paperwork, changing contacts, and elusive correspondence.

Like Miss Clavel in the timeless children's book *Madeline*, I began to have a hunch that "something was not right." The simple fact that there might be more than one social service agency handling Early Intervention cases in New York City or that some of those agencies might be better equipped for Eden wouldn't have occurred to me. So it was just a lucky coincidence that one of my friends had a friend whose job was to help parents like me, parents who needed to navigate a logistically daunting territory for their children. I never met this friend of a friend in person, but over the phone she assured me that I wasn't without options. There were several Early Intervention agencies, and some were known for having especially skilled therapists and administrators. With her advice, I reopened Eden's bursting medical folder and began the paperwork to file his case with a new social service agency. I was the recipient of timely generosity.

Eden was about nineteen months old by the time his case was handled by a second agency. By then I could see that therapy, like Eden's medical care, was recognizable as right. Right for him. And lo, Eden's third social worker, Stacey, quietly and competently assembled a mini all-star team. Team Eden.

Stacey's timing compounded my gratitude. I was in the middle of learning how to manage Eden's particular needs. As a child with special health needs, Eden was one among ten million American children. His intensive eczema care regimen and dietary rules certainly seemed doable compared with monitoring insulin levels, pushing a wheelchair, or attending to children who cannot use a toilet, and I understood the relativity of children's special needs. Still, I continued to get overwhelmed.

A simple routine offers an illustration. Doctor Anderson wanted me to soak Eden up to his neck for twenty to thirty minutes daily. Those soaks saturated his skin cells with moisture, and the lotion I patted all over him sealed it in. Half an hour is a long time for a child that young to stay engaged in near flotation. In those early evenings of summer I sat in our steamy bathroom on the closed toilet or on the floor, with my bottom sinking into an old couch cushion to spare my coccyx. Thus positioned, I alternately arranged mosaics of plastic on the tiling and read aloud from puffy plastic bath books. Eden's favorite plot line involved a mouse named Maisy who was perpetually interrupted during her bath until one of her friends jumped in with her; frankly, that felt disturbingly suggestive on my side of that porcelain tub. *Don't get any ideas, buddy . . .*

When Eden tired and fussed to come out early, I brought in kitchen utensils—ladles, spatulas, pots, kettles, and the like. He particularly liked the streams that poured through the bottom of pasta colanders with measuring spoons trapped behind. Eden played with everything offered as long as I played too. My eyelids grew heavy in our urban rain-forest mist. When Eden saw my head rolling toward my collarbone, he splashed his objections. My head would jerk up in response, and as my left hand twisted to expose my watch, my right one grabbed the nearest spoon to "stir the soup" for five more minutes. I had been literally and figuratively carrying Eden so long that he didn't understand flying solo. That was where Team Eden came to us, flexing its collective muscle.

Team Eden consisted of three therapists from the New York League for Early Learning Lifestart program. First came Charlotte. She was Eden's feeding and occupational therapist. Why would a child need therapy to learn to eat? Isn't eating instinctive? Nope. Not if your food has been going in the wrong direction practically from the first swallow. His pattern of vomiting had created a sensory memory, meaning that his food often came up his throat as a reflex. Pediatric feeding therapy is used to treat physical or behavioral feeding obstacles like Eden's.

I would also learn that children who have had a history of "disrupted eating" tend to adapt behaviors such as overstuffing their mouths to locate their food and preferring particularly "safe"-feeling food textures. *Safe* is different for every child. I have a friend whose son would eat only mushy soft foods because he didn't have normal muscle tone in his throat. Eden favored hard, dry food because he could feel where his chewed pretzels were as they moved through his mouth and throat; he could control the process.

Charlotte was a puppet master. With her frosted blond hair, hourglass figure, and Texas accent, she confidently fed Eden as if dicing and spooning pears were part of her Southern female birthright. Good thing. Her job daunted me, and Eden knew it. I dreaded when he gagged on food made and offered by my hand. Instead, Charlotte confidently zoomed right in on my source of that dread: Eden's mouth. Every time she came, he ate.

She portioned bites of food into the correct shapes and sizes. She counted slowly while he labored to swallow liquid. "We're gettin' all the way to four today, my friend!" she would drawl.

They chitchatted! At first Charlotte didn't get a lot of small talk from Eden. At one and a half years old, he was stuck in one- and two-word combinations, and he didn't have many. He made up words for some familiar objects, like calling his hamburgers "Ana." But Charlotte continued to beam her sky-blue eyes into his and gently prod, "C'mon, my friend. Just look what I've got for you today!" Charlotte made meals into a wonderland with sparkly utensils, twirled straws, novelty toothpicks, and plastic toy gadgets for Eden to play with between bites. Those gadgets didn't just distract him from his efforts; Eden began to commit his small muscles to toys that gratified with sound and motion, continuing both his fine and gross motor development. Charlotte believed that once Eden felt comfortable chewing and swallowing, he would become less sensitive overall.

Over time, Eden opened his mouth to the foods that previously had signaled danger: slippery bits of grapes or rice milk with all sorts of thickening purees. He still choked on occasion, but less often. When he did, Charlotte pulled both of us into a safe zone.

"I don't know; he just threw up his bread all over himself this morning, and now he's fine. Maybe my bread is too soft," I fretted one afternoon.

"He is fine, just *fine*." She blazed her blue eyes at me. "We just need to keep on using those throat muscles. All the kids do that. Let's keep an eye on that bread. I'll give him some tomorrow."

One day, while the three of us sat at the table nibbling cut fruit, I was telling Charlotte that one of Eden's doctors had recommended he have an endoscopy, but we had looked for other opinions. Charlotte remarked, "I had a client whose GI wanted her baby's feeding tube reinserted instead of trying to feed. But I worked that baby through it. No tube, just patience. You know, that mother said to me, 'These GIs! They make their recommendations, and then they go home and have dinner with their family. I go home and I eat my heart out.'" Charlotte shook her head in a swift pantomime of maternal frustration.

"Isn't that right? Isn't that just right?" she asked, turning back to me with a squint. She recognized me as that mother too.

There were two other therapists on Team Eden. One was a speech therapist named Pam. Pam had a big black rolling suitcase filled with toys and books, like a year-round Santa Claus. For the first few months, Pam was simply a teacher who could find two hundred things to do with one wooden car puzzle, a pleasant woman who happened to look like my mother-in-law, a weekly visitor who appreciated and drank a glass of ice water and often asked for another. Then, one special day, she received my junior high school title of "cool" and became Pam Who Rocks the Casbah. That was the day she rushed out of the bedroom five minutes early, red-faced and nearly bursting: "You *cannot* believe what your son said to me today!"

It seemed Pam had asked Eden, as she had every single session, what he had eaten for lunch. Instead of answering literally, Eden had answered with a knowing glint: "I ate Pam for lunch." Humor. He had *joked*. Whether it was funny didn't matter to Pam. She understood that a mother who has spent days or even hours in a vacuum of anxiety feels disproportionate joy in her child's display of the ordinary, and she rejoiced with me.

The last therapist to join Team Eden was a physical therapist (PT) named Mathew. Eden had rolled and sat up in a timely manner during his first year, but the months that followed his first birthday had been disrupted by his allergies. Our arms and his stroller had provided his mobility. Eden began walking at about nineteen months, an innocuous tardiness if it were not for his health history. Mathew was assigned to build up Eden's muscle strength and, as important, his confidence. How? By playing big muscle games. (FYI, mothers: The next time the father of your children starts tossing one of them around over his head, think twice before you fret over safety and tender tummies. The "airplane's comin' in for landing!" game boosts physicality and abdominal strength.)

Honestly, for me, the allure of the playground had rusted with years of use, and I was worn. I wished I were more like those mothers who Pied Pipered impromptu hopscotch tournaments, with children flocking behind them to join. And I paled in comparison with the Sunday daddies, the "isn't this great, buddy, I just love getting out into the fresh air with my kid, let's play ball, buddy" fathers who work outside the home all week. Question: Why do the Sunday daddies seem so energetic? Answer: Because they are *Sunday* daddies.

In fact, when Dayna was a playground toddler, Drew and I referred to one such Sunday daddy as Absentee Father. Not because we saw him only on Sundays but because he always brought at least half a dozen rambunctious children and the entire Sunday *New York Times*, a hopeful but futile prop he scanned, at best, while standing strategically between the sandbox and the climbing bars. Meanwhile, his children accosted their peers, vividly illustrating the Darwinian truth that what Dad didn't see made them stronger. We joked that Dad wouldn't have been bothered if the children were doing bong hits out of their bubble blowers.

Drew and I swapped endless comments on Absentee Father's valiant attempts to ignore his aggressive children until one of his neighbors reported that he had only four children but all were under seven years old. (They moved so swiftly, it had looked like far more.) Furthermore, his wife worked long weekends, during which he was assigned full-time daddycare. Drew and I immediately stopped mocking him. God bless that father, we chimed. He may be as tired as we are.

Fortunately, Mathew, PT and PPP (professional playground pal), chose a career centered on children and, yes, playgrounds and kiddie gyms. To start, Eden didn't want to exert himself any more than grown-ups want to complete that ninth set of Pilates leg lifts. Whereas fitness aficionados want the flat abs seen on the screens of reality television, Eden had no such motivation. Mathew's challenge was keeping Eden engaged and willing to climb, pull, and jump.

When the playground became unbearably chilly, Mathew met us in a Tumbling Tots class and became Eden's personal trainer. At first glance, Mathew was a high-five, baseball cap kind of guy. As we began spotting Eden on the trampoline's side together, he revealed his studied interest in mind-body connections, nutrition, biochemistry, and philosophy. He had read countless books on those topics and even brought me some to read. As a result, when I heard Mathew chirp for the thousandth time, "Uppie Puppy!" as Eden's short legs swung under the parallel bars, I sensed that the man underneath my son was graced with a mind as vigorous as his body. Eden's therapists made me remember something. As a child I had a dance teacher who wore the expected clingy black tunics and quoted aloud, "You must always remember, girls. Dance is what happens *between* the steps." Eden's therapists exemplified my teacher's refrain: They could have just choreographed Eden. Instead, their love persuaded him to take on the high leaps and spins.

In fact, when Team Eden first entered our lives, I can mark just how off course we had gone. Back in the month of July 2004, a few days before I met Charlotte, our living room floorboards were flooded from a leak underneath. When the boards began to buckle slightly, I wiped the wet areas with paper towels and assumed they would flatten again. A few days later I stubbed the tops of all five toes walking to the coffee table. Pulling up the living room area carpet, I gawked. There were smooth bumps nearly six inches high growing under the carpet; there had been a water leak from a nearby apartment.

Somehow another day passed before I remembered to alert our building manager. The bumps became molehills. Then three of the formations grew to eight inches high and another one sprouted. Problem was, it was Friday and repairpersons couldn't get there until the next Tuesday. Over the weekend the floor swelled with abandon. One bump came nearly to my midthigh. Monday afternoon, Dayna entertained herself by standing atop the tallest one, wearing a gold-embroidered yarmulke, waving a wand, and shouting, "I'm king of the mountain!"

When I opened our front door to Charlotte, I made a joke about some "motor-physical sensory challenges" in our living room, sort of sensing the strange scene with Dayna prancing about like a riled-up billy goat. But in truth those random three-foot swells erupting from the floor jibed nicely with my inner landscape. Nothing felt normal at that time, and so normality would have been more cause for notice or concern. After the boards were replaced the next day, I completely forgot about them.

Eden met all his Early Intervention goals at the same time he "aged out" at three years old, about a year and a half after our bizarre floor swelling. Eden hadn't had any long-term intrinsic sensory issues; his body had just been too overloaded with physical discomfort during his earliest years. Sounds simple, yet Drew and I could have talked ourselves into believing that he would simply outgrow his issues as others had assured us.

One fine day, a few months after we had expressed our heartfelt good-byes to Team Eden, Drew, Dayna, Eden, and I went walking along the East River to the playground in Carl Schurz Park. The air was dry and so clear that I could see a jogger rounding the tip of Roosevelt Island halfway toward the shore of Queens. Dayna and Eden walked ahead, bikes and strollers passing them. They wanted to see the big dogs chase one another in the fenced-in dog park. It was all dust and dogs and flying pebbles, but Dayna and Eden had learned to love the press of their faces against the metal fence and the involuntary jump when the big dogs came close.

I stumbled over a piece of cracked cement on the river walk and looked down. The gray slating was jutting up into an arch, broken bits of cement around it, as if punched from underneath. "Yikes!" I turned to Drew.

But I didn't really see Drew. I saw those buckled floorboards. And then I looked ahead at Eden and measured nothing more complicated than his happiness against the time line they had commenced. It had been a steady rise since then. Now Eden couldn't wait to see those dogs. He broke into a run, wispy blond hair flapping and glinting in the sun, arms flung straight behind him like the wings of a fighter plane extended for takeoff. His muscular thin legs pumped with increasing speed underneath a stiff upright torso. Chest thrust out, he sped forward, wildly grinning. We didn't call out. We let him go.

"He thinks he really can fly, you know," Drew said slowly.

"He can," I answered. "Now he can."

And then, as Dayna chased her brother into the East River wind, I saw them—Charlotte, Pam, and Mathew. Their arms were forever outstretched.

Chapter 4

SWORD FIGHTING TO MUZAK

THE FIRST TIME IT HAPPENED, I was twirling spaghetti. The excitement had peaked at Dayna's spaghetti lunch. It was an annual preschool custom in which the children prepared the pasta, the parents arrived carrying shopping bags of desserts, and then everyone feasted together in the church refectory. Dayna, mute from pleasure, ate three plates of spaghetti while sauce dripped down the front of her periwinkle jumper until, like the rest of the children, she was sated by the grouping of beloved people and carbs. She excused herself from our table to jump out her excitement. I watched as she and her classmates discovered old tree trimmings on the stage and began twirling them above their heads.

That was when I felt it: a strange certainty that I wasn't there. I didn't feel invisible; I felt gone. I had gone somewhere else even if no one could see it. I could still see the children and parents, all the activity around me, but I couldn't get to it. I'm sure only a few minutes passed as I sat in my folding chair watching the children play as if through a glass pane. On the other side there was the savory aroma of bottled red sauce on coil heaters, mothers smiling and cocking their heads to keep their offspring in view, teachers nibbling at the underbaked Pillsbury chocolate chip cookies that left sugar granules on the tongue, and children shrieking with the certainty that they could, and would, shriek. Crowded as the other side was, I was the only person on my side of the glass, the sounds and smells leaking faintly through.

Then the reprimand: "Children! No more playing with the tinsel!" And I was back. Just like that. The feeling had passed. I shrugged it off as mental fatigue. After all, exhaustion had become dangerously familiar because Eden, at one and a half, was awake every night like a soldier in a foxhole. Deep into the darkness, I grabbed toward the shadows, sang, and fetched water and blankets.

In the weeks before the spaghetti lunch, I restocked and relabeled the pantry; reapplied to a second social service agency; purchased extra medical emergency kits; and designed a new filing system with folders labeled "Allergy Product Information," "Eden's Health Records I, II, and III," and "Allergy Updates." I enrolled Dayna in swimming classes and sat poolside scribbling the dates and appearances of Eden's recent reactions into my spiral purse-size notebook, putting double asterisks next to some of the words: "**Honeydew one slight hive" or "Stye in left eye, park but no sandbox." Despite more than a year of chronically interrupted sleep, I had tapped into adrenaline that I used to fuel our allergic new life.

How had I managed to defy the biological relationship between fatigue and energy? Easy. Caffeine! Lots of it. I drank carefully calibrated doses of coffee both inside and outside my apartment. My surrounding sidewalks were rife with options, and I became the neighborhood junkie.

I favored two nearby delis on First Avenue. New York delis have the unique advantage of adhering to the New York coffee code. In delis I didn't need to contend with soy, foam, syrup, or Italian vocabulary. I had to but mutter, "Coffee regular, please" (a splash of milk and one stirred sugar packet), and seconds later I held my happy blue cardboard cup with an etching of the Acropolis. I slurped at those cups with abandon, the jagged tears on the plastic lids pleasantly scraping my upper lip.

In a pinch, the small fruit store on 88th Street had a self-serve coffee kiosk next to a counter piled with dried-out fig bars and aging muffins. In a tighter time pinch and directly across our street there was a vending stand that Drew referred to as the roach coach. Stacks of prebuttered bagels and pastries were held captive by a display dusted with stale sticky particles. The sugar doughnuts looked as if they had run up against the glass Wile E. Coyote–style until flattened. I tried to be more discerning, but I was a busy mother.

I had many justifications for my addiction (coffee is healthier than soda . . . sort of . . . just until both kids are in school . . . new research shows coffee prevents Alzheimer's and I *really* need to stay sharp . . .). But my strongest defense was that I needed as much time as possible to compile a freakish kind of food knowledge. These were the kinds of obscure nutritional facts that parents and caretakers of children with food allergies, celiac disease, diabetes, Crohn's disease, and the like, need to know for their children's safety. It was storehouse information that required something like a photographic memory alongside the nocturnal rhythms of a teenager.

Eden's food allergy diagnosis wasn't timed advantageously in respect to available information about food safety and ingredients. Then again, is there a good time to develop life-threatening allergies? We learned about his allergies in the winter of 2003–2004, a year plus before food-labeling laws took effect. Eventually, the Food Allergen Labeling and Consumer Protection Act of 2004 mandated that food products containing milk, eggs, fish, crustacean shellfish, peanuts, tree nuts, wheat, and soy must identify those foods (the eight most common allergens) in plain language on the ingredient list. Alternatively, the allergens must be listed via a parenthetical statement within the ingredient list or as an addendum after the ingredient list.

I learned about the Food Allergen Labeling and Consumer Protection Act months in advance in my monthly newsletter from the Food Allergy and Anaphylaxis Network. FAAN is a worldwide food allergy and anaphylaxis advocacy organization that I joined after Eden's diagnosis, and I've relied on it for food allergy information and education for years. As excited as I was about the new law, it took awhile for the food industry to revise all those labels, and I filled that time silently deciphering ingredients in food stores. I remember an internal debate about the safety of Nestlé cocoa powder. The ingredients were "cocoa powder." Hmm. So I compared the powder label to the label on Nestlé Toll House Chocolate Chips (an item I knew I wasn't supposed to feed Eden). On the latter, milk was listed last. My thought process went like this: *Okay, maybe they add milk to the chips after the powder is added, or maybe they don't use the cocoa powder to make the chips but maybe the powder is run on the same equipment as the hot chocolate mix, which does have a lot of milk in it.*

Now there are iPhone applications and computer programs that have been created for food allergies that tally, analyze, chart, and compare macro and micro ingredients for parents like me. There has been so much progress. In fact, in September 2008, the U.S. Food and Drug Administration (FDA) even held a public hearing on the use of advisory "may contain" labeling on packaged food items. In other words, the labeling on a box of cookies can easily read "May contain tree nuts and peanuts" without having those ingredients listed, and that can be fairly confusing. Most parents of allergic children simply bypass items that "may contain" their child's allergens. However, the FDA is developing a long-term strategy to help manufacturers use these statements more clearly.

But by late spring 2004 I couldn't learn fast enough. If invited, I would have happily donned a hairnet to inspect a General Mills factory. I spent hours of screen time cruising through parenting sites and blogs, where I learned about the controversy regarding corn syrup solids and the allergic possibilities of seemingly safe bread products (egg-washed crusts, wayward seeds, contaminated equipment; let me count the ways). I researched preservatives I had no intention of allowing on our shelves *just in case*. "Hmmm. Inert lactose might be safe, but sodium lactate sounds dicey because it can be derived from milk as well as fruit sugars," I mumbled at Drew while we sat at our dining room table, shuffling through bills.

On the way down to the laundry room, I interrogated my Orthodox neighbor on subtle implications of the Kosher D symbol. I built silos of information in the aisles of supermarkets, dizzy under the spell of the piped-in Muzak. I startled when the intercom bleated, "He-elp in produce!"

Somewhere in those aisles, I had begun my personal quest. Scrutinizing box after box of crackers and cereals wasn't just a means to a new way of eating; it was one more means to keep my child alive. Whereas other mothers fretted over refined flours, my anxiety was practically limitless and was at times nearly electric. It shifted from palpable terror to petty grievance to life to whole grains to absorbable calcium, reaching finally to death. Like a tightrope walker, I kept my gaze forward because if I looked down at the possibilities, surely I would fall.

When I look back on my state of mind, it's not surprising how often I met with hurt and anger. To be clear—mine. Like the rainy Sunday morning when Dinosaur Boy's parents came to our home for the first and last time. A few months earlier Dayna and a boy had bonded over his plastic dinosaurs at the playground. After a few weeks of Dayna enjoying the company of Michael, aka Dinosaur Boy (Dayna was probably Chalk Pail Girl), his mother, Lorraine, asked me to exchange phone numbers for playdates. We arranged one or two playground meetings before taking the next step and breaking bread.

Or, bagels, as it turned out. Like Dayna, Michael was bored the Sunday morning I called for a playdate. Lorraine jumped on my invitation, promptly offering, "I'll bring bagels and stuff."

Her generosity sent me flying into the kitchen to bake a mock bagel for Eden. Mock bagels had become one of my staple foods thanks to instant-rise yeast and Eden's ignorance of authentic New York bagels. At least mine looked authentic. Or so I thought.

An hour later, with toys and costumes strewn about the living room, I invited Lorraine and her husband, Steve, to their chairs and popped into the kitchen, where Drew was supposed to be finding coffee mugs. Instead his arm was swirling the countertops in frantic circles, sponging poppy seeds as if Eden would be entering at any moment to lick the Formica clean. Sighing, I redirected Drew to the silverware drawer, brought Eden's bagel to his booster seat, and settled Dayna and Michael at the kid table with Dixie cups of apple juice.

Then I sat.

"Oh!" Lorraine popped the word like a balloon. "That's so cute! Oh!" Another pop. "Is *that*," she said, pointing at Eden's plate, "because of his allergies?"

"Yeah, I bake his things just to be safe." I was intentionally vague because too much detail predictably steered conversation toward a lengthy analysis of the list.

Satisfied, Lorraine nodded. Then, most delicately, she picked up a piece of smoked salmon that had dropped from her bagel to her plate and rearranged it atop her sliced tomato, pushing into the orange flesh with her pointer finger. I had profane thoughts about the fish oils.

Bagel raised in midair, Lorraine brought her stare back to Eden. "But look at him. He eats so well. He always eats everything you give him!" Her head swiveled toward Steve. "Susan gives him hamburger in the playground!"

"Wow," said Steve, lifting a piece of cantaloupe into his mouth, eyes averted.

I breathed in through my nose, praying that Steve's monosyllabic response would end Lorraine's observations. But no, Lorraine bent toward me, a misleading posture considering that her next remark was broadcast in high volume. "Michael is so picky! He won't eat turkey or chicken or anything green or even eggs. He only ever wants muffins and bread. At least when you feed Eden, you know that's all he can have. At least you know you don't have any other choice! Keep it simple, am I right?"

Right.

Her remark resonated for days after. *You don't have any other choice!* Of course she didn't mean for me to feel pleased with Eden's allergies, and of course she was probably trying to find the proverbial silver lining. But at that time my nerves were too raw for platitudes. I didn't want to talk food with anyone except Drew and Eden's doctors. Yet educating the people around Eden was part of my new job as the parent of an allergic child.

Indeed, in the summer of 2004, Eden's second summer, that glass began to come down more often, a window that shut before I knew I was even looking through it. One particularly lousy afternoon, the sprinkler drain in our playground clogged overnight. The result inspired Dayna to linger in the rarefied tepid gray slosh. After a while Eden began steeping in anxious exhaustion. He was and still is a hot little guy. I pushed his stroller around the perimeter of the park until he finally fell into a silent sleep, both of us beaded in sweat.

That was when Dayna announced that she had "to pee can't wait Mommy quick!" In the doorless public bathroom, as I jerked the stroller back and forth, the other forearm propping Dayna's stall door open, Eden's moist skull rose in acute comprehension of his circumstances. His wails echoed off stained walls that smelled exactly like the twenty years of acrid urine they enclosed.

When we finally got back to the bench for a quick hand wiping before the walk home, two mothers with their little boys strolled over. One of them whined when his mother handed him a granola bar. In politically correct modern mom fashion she gently passed it back to him, saying, "Okay, I hear you, Joshie. Maybe just one bite." Then she turned to her friend, eyebrows raised. "He doesn't like this kind very much, but it's healthy. These days I eschew all hydrogenated oils. I just *won't*, you know? It's too important."

Slam! The wall was down. I stewed in hate. Oh, *yes*. Yes. Hydrogenated oils are so important. Important enough to *eschew*! I slumped like an adolescent and cast furtive daggers at those mothers. But I knew they fell short since those women didn't deserve my enmity. So I moved away. Unfair. Still. Unfair that I no longer had their luxury. *I* wanted to worry about hydrogenated oils. I wanted to belong to their club.

On the way home, I felt ashamed for my inability to cope with the situation and an overheard remark. How I was going to find a way to tolerate comments like theirs? I said stuff like that before Eden. I had all sorts of self-imposed rules back when I freely fed my first child, just like those mothers who could pick their own food battles instead of playing interpreter to every biological symptom and cereal box label.

Crisis sometimes felt like an easier position to assume than normality. I showed flashes of certainty and verve during Eden's weekly minicrises. A sudden flair of eczema, a pronounced gag on canned corn—those were my moments. I rose to those occasions. Even as Eden's emotional and physical health slowly improved, I felt like I was parenting on steroids, with an energy that consumed me.

Our new doorwoman greeted me at the end of that afternoon. She buzzed intercoms to warn residents of their dinners, stacked in plastic bags and insulated, pungent valises in the arms of deliverymen who would bring them up the service elevator. "Good evening!" rang in an endless background loop. Although I often longed for privacy within the thrum of my populated lifestyle, that evening the three of us might as well have been urban castaways marooned in a thirty-floor co-op. I might have banished myself to one side of the world entirely if not for my children. I didn't want them to have to keep me company.

Later, after lights out for Dayna and Eden, I took the phone and myself under the throw blanket of my bed and called my friend Coleen. Coleen and I met in ninth grade on the first day of school. Within a week of high school we had learned everything about each other that could possibly matter. We spent the next four years quelling our age-appropriate anguish, smoking the occasional cigarette, and squinting into tirades of complaints about our undeserving parents. Now Coleen was a mother of two and contented in her career. Nonetheless, she came from a large Irish Catholic family with the accompanying angst. Their occasional bouts of despair seemed genetic, along with small noses and lightly freckled legs. I knew that Coleen had become somewhat versed on therapies by way of familial osmosis.

"Depression is when everything seems like too much effort, when everything feels too hard to even begin," she said. "Do you feel like you can't get out of bed in the morning? Are you crying uncontrollably?"

"No. On both counts." I was equally confident. "I cry once in a while when Drew and I argue over stupid stuff like who forgot to say 'good morning.' But I don't want to go on medication. There's been too much medicine in our house already." I elaborated: "I feel like I can be a great mom as long as something is clearly wrong with Eden but not when I just have to be a normal parent. I'm always second-guessing myself or wishing things were different. I want to make things feel right, however they have to be. I'm worried medication will just make me feel less like myself. You know?"

"Well," she began, "I mean, I remember that time after 9/11 when I was so stressed and just took something for a week. It helped so much. That was so nice." She paused at the recollection. "But if not, maybe you should talk to someone who has experience with families . . . like yours?" She said she would ask around.

Instead, within the next few weeks, another close friend suggested a Doctor Reiss. "I didn't use her, but a good friend—remember Marie? She said she was great after her divorce." She paused again. "And I think Doctor Reiss has a grown daughter with a medical something. I'm honestly not sure what."

After I hung up I reviewed what I knew about therapists: when people mentioned their therapists in passing, though articulate enough they didn't seem that much more able to solve their problems. My parents had occasionally referred to the world of therapy in conversations. In fact, my mother used to roll words like *psychosomatic* and *repressed* around her tongue like hard candy. "I have a psychosomatic dislike for tea," she would explain. "My mother made me drink it when I was sick, so it triggers negative memories."

I didn't know how I felt about therapy. I wasn't against it, but I was overloaded. I didn't want therapy-speak cluttering my thoughts. And then there was the time commitment. We had just put together Team Eden, and we had appointments with his developmental therapists all week long. Why make life more complicated? My predicament was simple. I didn't feel *normal*. Everything had changed with Eden, yet that very fact was inexplicable, too dramatic for me. Then how to feel ordinary? The smallest decisions fell under the gloom of that question. I kept thinking about attending a support group for parents like me, but what if doing so made me feel even more alone? What if the other allergy parents didn't feel the way I did? It felt like a risk, though I would learn it wasn't. In a 2006 survey conducted of eighty-seven families of children with food allergies, 41 percent of the parents reported increased feelings of stress related to their children's condition.[11] I called Doctor Reiss, hoping to find my normal without even entertaining the possibility that my anxiety was normal. It just wasn't helpful.

Five years after my first conversation with Doctor Reiss, the Food Allergy Initiative, an organization devoted to, among other things, conducting research toward finding a cure and improving the quality of life for food-allergic individuals, would conduct a study that examined "caregivers' quality of life" as it relates to food allergies. The study, conducted from 2008 to 2009, found that a lower quality of life is significantly more likely among caregivers who "have a child who had been to the emergency department for food allergy in the past year; have a child with multiple food allergies; are more knowledgeable about food allergies; have a child who is allergic to milk, wheat, or egg—possibly because these allergies tend to affect young children and/or because avoiding these foods 'requires more vigilance and therefore more anxiety' than avoiding peanuts."[12]

Over the phone I told Doctor Reiss, "My son has been sick from food allergies, and even though he isn't really anymore, I think that maybe enough things have happened to me that I need to talk to someone about it all." After I hung up, I spent several minutes wondering what other people say the first time they call a therapist.

When I met Doctor Reiss, my eyes were drawn to her shoes. They were brown, shapely, possibly Danish, walking sandals. Since my footwear had been reduced to anything capable of holding up under pavement-pounding miles, I imagined myself in a similar pair, hoping my envy was a good sign. Imitation is a sign of flattery, or how did it go? Her frizzy graying hair grazed her shoulders by an inch, and her smile was wide but not lingering.

Her office had rows of books lining built-in shelves to the ceiling and a plastic framed print of Matisse's *Lady in Blue* on the wall over her couch. We sat in wide, soft reclining chairs in front of a couch. As we faced each other from the safety of our brown enclaves, I wondered who went first.

Doctor Reiss did. She asked me, "Do you want to tell me what happened?" That was the only question she asked me that day.

I began when Eden was inside me. That was our beginning, my first bodily communication with my child, his head leaning into my ribs and his movements slow. I fully expected Doctor Reiss to push me ahead to the important part—Eden's allergies—just when, unexpectedly, there was so much else I needed to tell her.

I told her how sure I was my second turn at mothering would be both easy and awesome. And I had planned to teach part time. And I had seen myself striking a balance between parenting and my professional commitments. I told her that when I thought about the other teachers, I missed them, missed being a part of something besides my family, and at the same time, I wanted to be close to Eden as he healed mentally and physically. And finally I told her that despite evidence to the contrary, I wondered if I had missed some crucial moment when I could have prevented Eden's allergic landslide if only I had known that was the moment.

She listened. Doctor Reiss listened to my pauses and to my retractions. She listened with her face, and then she leaned in and listened with her skin. With her alert, sixty-watt eyes, she pulled me into a sunbath of compassion. And who knew I would turn out to be a pushover, an open-legged therapy slut? By the end of our session I was sobbing with relief. For that one hour, I hardly cared that orgasmic confessions wouldn't solve my anxieties.

But during the two weeks that passed until our next appointment, questions arose from day to day and I promised myself to ask them. *This therapy business needs to be worth its time.* During my second session, Doctor Reiss told me that her daughter had a life-threatening allergy to antibiotics and other medicines. *Hmm. Let's see.* I still wasn't ready to believe that her experience qualified her to help me with mine. I asked, "Well, then, I wanted to bring something up. So, uh, it's not like Eden can really talk yet, he's not even two, but I need to tell him *something* when he sees me or Dayna or Andrew eating what he can't have."

I shrugged. "I don't want to tell him 'when he's older' because that may be a lie. I don't want to scare him and tell him he'll be sick, and anyway 'sick' is different. I know that kids have faced worse deprivations than not getting to try their sister's pancakes but . . ."

I trailed off. *Am I missing something? Am I making it all too hard?*

She pushed her unruly hair behind her ears. "Other children's deprivations aren't really the point. Not for a child that young. And *older* and *sick* are too abstract for him anyway. Eden can only understand something concrete at his age. He knows the word *itchy?*" She tilted her head.

"I think so. He points at his eczema. He knows it's there." Truthfully, I wasn't sure.

"Fine. So you say, 'Eden, that will make you itchy.' And pantomime scratching with your hand as you say it." She held up one arm and pretended to scratch at it with her opposite hand. "He'll accept that answer." She spoke with finality. That was that.

Too simple. I didn't believe her.

The next day, during a calm weekday breakfast, Eden pointed at Dayna's cereal bowl, which of course was her favorite honey *nut* flavored variety. And Eden asked, "Haf that?"

Unquestionably off-pitch, I answered, "Eden, that will make you itchy." I even did the scratch mime. Eden looked at me for as long as a twenty-month-old can hold a stare and went back to silently chewing squares of toast.

I began to trust that Doctor Reiss could help me talk about allergies to Eden and maybe even the rest of the world. She reminded me of the things I knew but always forgot: Eden was at an exhausting age for any parent. Period. Sleep was important. I needed to slow down my pace and try to get more of it. Drew too. The two of us were so tired, we had taken to pulling at each other's patience with the masochistic pleasure of peeling sunburned skin off our own flesh. We kept forgetting that we didn't have to solve every puzzle of Eden's allergies every day. In fact, if I could offer families newly diagnosed with food allergies only one single piece of advice, it would be similar to the Alcoholics Anonymous mantra of "one day at a time." Drew and I harbored vexing allergy-related images of Eden as a teenager, a college student, or a groom eating his wedding cake. "How will he ever go to sleepaway camp?" we asked each other. Such thoughts only distracted us from solving Eden's needs as a toddler.

As with any good therapist, the other half of having Doctor Reiss was that she was a place where I could safely tell my stories. Like the story of the day a toddler spilt his nacho-flavored Doritos into the sandbox. Everyone stared while I jumped up from the cement border to lure Eden to a different spot with my fake happy face and red shovel. As their eyes followed me, my unease surrounded me like the sadness that rose in my stomach every morning when I woke.

There was the story of Eden's death. The point in every single day when I worried not *just* about Eden dying but about when or where I might think about Eden dying. I dreaded the uncertainty of all these imaginings because they occurred anywhere and without warning. I thought about him dying in checkout lines, in the kitchen, and when he woke up in the night. And in the night, even after I was back in bed listening to Eden shuffle around, I couldn't stop. I blamed Drew because he insisted on the monitor's top volume, just in case, and that was of course code for the unspeakable. And so Drew and I skirted any mention of Eden's death because we didn't know how else to go about our days, how to brush our teeth and check our e-mail in the same life where we openly acknowledged our son's medical odds.

And then there was the problem of not wanting to be me. I told Doctor Reiss that once when I walked with Dayna and Eden down the summertime streets, we passed a single outdoor diner leaning over a square white plate of charred asparagus. In the moments that followed, I thought about this stranger for too long. I wondered how he might have spent his morning and whether that man in the blue silk tie had ever felt what I was hiding. Did blue-tie man ever feel tired in his veins and bone marrow? And had he ever grown tired of himself? Did his white wine taste as feathery and cool as it looked? I imagined pushing the chair back from that table and going to his home inside his body instead of mine.

Doctor Reiss grasped it all—my leaden anxiety and my mundane annoyances. None of my stories were too large or small for her. I could leave her office with that much less to contend with. Doctor Reiss didn't give me therapy-speak, but she gave definition to my shapeless feelings. She identified the episodes I have been having since Spaghetti Lunch as "dissociation." It is a sense of detachment from the reality around you.

"You're not going to keep feeling that way forever," Doctor Reiss assured me. "You've got a tremendous amount of anxiety on your plate, no pun intended. More than average. You know for sure that your child *can* flatline. It's going to pull you out at times, along with some anger. Trust me. You just have to learn how to get back. That's what we do together."

In the years to come, long after I stopped seeing Doctor Reiss on a regular basis, she would continue to be a resource for me and for Drew. He and I visited the doctor together a handful of times when we felt confused about handling Eden's anxieties. We would ask her for school strategies for Eden or for ways to make ourselves more comfortable advocating for him.

But then, as I felt the anchor of Doctor Reiss's advice, I also felt a new curiosity about the whole story of allergies—the big beast lurking behind me. So I ordered a few used books on Amazon. I read that allergies were old but Eden's multiple and anaphylactic variety was new. The term *allergy* was coined in 1906, but the condition has been recognized since ancient times. As far back as the fourth century BC, the Greek physician Hippocrates recorded the contradiction that some generally healthy and nourishing foods made a few people sick.

In 95 BC, the Roman philosopher and poet Lucretius wrote in his famous scientific poem *On the Nature of Things* that what was good for some might be poison for others. I still think about this when I encounter an extreme health food faddist who tries to convince me that Eden would be fine "if only . . ." I have learned that there are people who cannot believe that what they consider healthy is not healthy for everyone. These people tell me that if *only* I had given Eden raw as opposed to pasteurized milk or put him on a particular diet involving hemp seeds and dried seaweed, his life would be different.

By the mid-sixteenth century, allergic reactions to the environment were getting widely noticed in Europe. There were several recorded reports of rose fever, or what we call hay fever. And an Italian physician treated the Archbishop of Edinburgh for asthma in 1552 by instructing the clergyman to remove all the feathers from his bedding.

Then in 1819, a London physician, John Bostock, described a seasonal nose infection that was dubbed Bostock's summer catarrh. An English scientist named Charles Blackley, who had an asthma attack, possibly from a vase of dried grasses, built upon Bostock's observations. When he scratched the grass pollen into his skin, the resulting inflammation proved that pollen could cause an allergic reaction.

Later, in 1906, Clemens Peter Freiherr von Pirquet, an Austrian scientist and pediatrician, noticed a pattern in some of his young patients who had quick and severe reactions to vaccines. He, along with Bela Schick, coined the word *allergy* from the Greek *allos* meaning "other" and *ergon* meaning "reaction." The big story: allergies are a reaction to the other. And now millions of children and adults are reacting against substances that should be tolerable but instead are biologically regarded as an other. That was our story.

With Eden and I in therapy, our household nearly an allergic rehab center, I made another ironic discovery: the stories about the relationship between allergies and psychology. One afternoon while the children and I were visiting my mother, I glanced at some photos on my mother's shelf and saw a book titled *Let's Have Healthy Children*.

Since my mother's books line the walls of her apartment like overgrown ivy, I wasn't surprised to see that it was published in the 1950s. The author, Adelle Davis, was a nutritionist whose reputation seemed to be split between a whole foods pioneer and questionable advice. Curious and charmed by the retro drawings, I brought the book home and read the chapter titled "What Can Be Done for Allergies."

Adelle Davis begins the chapter by asserting, "Most and probably all such conditions as reactions to foods, asthma, hay fever, eczema, hives and stuffy and drippy noses are in part or entirely, psychological in origin. They are largely caused by the fact that the emotional needs of the parents, particularly the mother, have not been met during their own childhood. Since these needs are unconscious, the parents, struggling to do their best are unaware of them. The allergy conditions, however, often clear up without any improvement in diet when the parents have had deep psychotherapy."[13]

Wait. I just need to clear up my deep-seated issues with my own mother and bingo, no more hives for Eden?

"Strawberries and cherries may remind a child of a nipple and cause him to relive some painful experience connected with nursing," I read on. "Chocolate and orange juice, because of color, may remind him of traumas associated with toilet training."[14]

While often off the wall, Ms. Davis's theories on allergies nagged at me. I kept digging around the Internet until I unearthed another infuriating tidbit. During the years from 1940 to 1959, Doctor M. Murray Peshkin, the medical director of the Children's Asthma Research Institute and Hospital in Denver, noticed that some of his most severe asthma patients improved markedly as soon as they were removed from their homes and hospitalized, but before their treatments had had a chance to work. Peshkin came to advocate *parentectomy*: a slang term that came to mean the removal of parents from a child. Peshkin believed that the childrens' symptoms were relieved by being away from allergens in their homes, and also their health improved during the separation from their parent, and any conflicts they might have had with them.

When I read a few lines to Drew, he asked, "Why are you spending your time on this idiocy? You know it's meaningless."

Of course Drew was right, and of course he was wrong. Those beliefs, though obscure and dated, weren't meaningless to me. Those texts were my proof of the history of disbelief surrounding Eden's allergies. And understanding that, in fact, helped me feel strangely grounded. *Imagine how misunderstood they must have felt—those other mothers.* I knew. I felt misunderstood even without provocation. Crazy, huh? Crazy, huh?

I came across Elliptical Woman by accident—a haggardly attractive brunette with half-moons under her eyes. She favored the elliptical machine next to mine when I eked out the time to go to my nearby gym. Why wasn't I using that time to get the rest Doctor Reiss advised? Not yet. When I lay down for naps, within minutes nervousness vibrated my eyelids open and the urgency of daylight pushed its way inside. Instead, I hoped this regular exercise would eventually recalibrate my hormones and force my body back to its pre-Eden rhythms.

The elliptical machines lulled me into hypnotic escape. Sneakers pushed snugly into pedals, fingers wrapped around handgrips, I backpedaled on the easiest manual course. It was easy to ignore the other women's exchanges: "Just hard-boiled eggs and green tea. That's it!" "It was so *cleansing*. I'll give you the number."

I don't know how I started a conversation with Elliptical Woman about our children's eating habits. I had trained myself to chitchat with mothers about anything else. But that day it felt okay to let her talk. I learned that Elliptical Woman gave her son smoothies with bananas and blueberries to disguise his daily fruit allotment. "He won't eat fruit, but he needs the vitamins."

Clever Elliptical Woman. How could I explain to this normal mother that my son was allergic to his first two baby formulas? That his throat muscles still rejected most liquids, bringing them up to remind me of all the wrong foods I allowed to go down? That he could not tolerate most fruits or that I had already tried making baby food blender drinks on his feeding therapist's suggestion? And anyway, who would want to drink a banana, Stage 1 pears, and formula shake? Eden certainly didn't. I avoided the elliptical machines the next gym session and began a new relationship with the Cybex climbing machines.

A few weeks later, I saw Elliptical Woman and her son in Barnes & Noble. I was with Eden, who was asleep in his stroller. Her little boy had disarmingly big brown bunny eyes, and although he looked to be at least six years old, he was grabbing every book off the shelf in front of him, one by one, and stacking them into piles of two, then four, then two again. He moved across the wide fields that lay between methodical and frantic. I allowed myself a guess. *Autistic.*

Elliptical Woman turned to me and said in one breath, "Do you come here a lot? I haven't seen you. We are always out, out somewhere, even in the winter, but then, he can't stay anywhere for very long. My mother always says to me, 'Why are you always running around so much? You look exhausted. He'll be all right, but you should sit down and drink one of those shakes yourself.' Anyway, I tell her, 'Ma, I can't stay in with him. I just can't.'"

She looked into me, and her gaze was not urgent like the daylight. It was the patient gaze of a near stranger who hoped I would meet her eyes. I did. And in her eyes I saw myself. I saw my guilt. I saw my irrational fear of connecting with other people and thus exposing Eden and myself. But also I saw myself healing. Slowly. But getting better nonetheless. More like her. Then I saw *her* relief. Confession over, she chased after her son into another aisle.

That night, as I was rinsing a plate while the water rose at the drain, the smoothies popped into mind. *Autistic kids have oral sensory issues too.* I remembered reading that thickened drinks and specific textures of food were recommended for autistic children. Just then, I knew her. Elliptical Woman was pumping and striding her way to her music, getting to the place where she did not supplicate to Velcro shoe bindings or dilute meds into grape juice. I knew the shadows on her face were dark love leaking through thin skin. She was jogging alongside the flurry of her own unexpected life with her child. She wasn't afraid to share it.

That day she joined my side, or maybe I joined hers. I believed that the specific backdrop of our lives didn't matter: "Even a trace of the wrong food could kill him." But it could have been "She's terrified of water" or "The tubes in his ears keep collapsing." Doesn't every mother at some point in her life fight tides of fear and shame? At some point we all may give our children the wrong cold medication, overprotect or underprotect, endure their petty humiliations, or make mistakes and worry that our children will suffer the consequences. Doesn't every mother flip the child-rearing book indexes, surf the Internet, try to click her way toward an answer when so often if she looked past the landscape of her heartbreak, she might see the hand of the woman treading the water beside her?

For over a year, friends and family had been offering up the names and stories of other parents. Everyone had known someone who knew someone: I had copied messages off my answering machine for months and ignored them, believing that no one could understand how I felt. "Susan, hi, listen, I have a friend . . ." "Oh, that sounds just like a little girl I met . . ." "There's this doctor I heard about . . ." I had business cards with phone numbers on the back. Scraps of paper: "I'll phone you." "E-mail me." "Call him."

Elliptical Woman unlocked me. She showed me that I wasn't going to get hurt if I called or e-mailed strangers or if I gave honest answers to the mothers who asked after Eden in school hallways. The least likely people offered resonating advice. A woman in New Hampshire, a friend of my cousin Lisa, happened to have a son whose list of allergic foods was almost identical to Eden's. After commiserating, she told me to stop heating Eden's food as soon as his next meal. "Serve it cold if you have to. It's crucial because you aren't going to have many packaged snacks as he gets older," she explained. "He needs to be okay with whatever temperature it is. You'll be bringing his food everywhere."

There was another mother who lived in Maryland, the daughter of my father's second wife's sister's brother-in-law's wife. Her child had a singular peanut allergy, and I spent most of the conversation silently envying the relative simplicity of her problem. Unlike me, she seemed to have her son's peanut allergy under control. I couldn't help but feel jealous, but that didn't mean she had it easier. Easier or harder wasn't the point. These conversations were about fear, though we parents never said it. And measuring and calculating my fears against theirs hadn't made me feel stronger; it had just made me feel lonely. I eventually learned that whether a conversation was satisfying or infuriating, whether the parent on the other side offered insight or silly platitudes, I wanted to be able to be *in* the conversation. That felt normal.

I wasn't alone. If a mother at Dayna's preschool told me she was up all night with her child, then that day I wasn't alone. If a father told me that his son fell onto the marble steps at the Museum of Natural History over the weekend because he wasn't holding his son's hand tightly enough and instead of seeing the dinosaurs, they spent the longest day of that man's life in the hospital, then I wasn't alone.

And just as all those realizations were coming to me, a mother showed me that if I kept it up, I wasn't just going to find company, I was going to be rewarded with *good* company. I never met Erin in person. She was a friend of a friend from Dayna's preschool. But we formed a fast phone friendship. I called her on the supposition that her son had Eden's kinds of allergies, though it turned out he didn't. However, he was Eden's age, and he wasn't growing.

The first time I spoke to Erin, she was operating under a theory that her son had multiple food intolerances. Her son had undergone two endoscopies and countless blood tests, had taken several kinds of stomach medications, and was enduring but not really eating an intricately customized diet of mung beans and millet. He had been premature, but even so, his lack of growth was very worrisome. Erin reported that he had chronic viruses and infections yet rarely fussed.

"He has pneumonia now, but you wouldn't know it," she tossed out.

So he really wasn't like Eden at all. Her son submitted silently to the exams, to the endless specialists all eagerly suggesting stomach medications and special diets to help him grow. "But he doesn't really eat anyway," Erin sighed one night as I cradled the phone against my armchair.

I could see him flicking food—chopped turkey and a few sprouted beans—around his plate, eyes darting elsewhere. It didn't matter that our sons were different. Separately, we had lived through days that were divided into periods of incremental unease, Mad Hatter tea parties of tension, weekends that devolved from family meals to snacks and stomachaches.

The next week Erin's son was going into the hospital for a hernia condition, which, she told me, wasn't an uncommon problem for preemies. I complimented her on her calm and described how decomposed Drew and I became at similar prospects. We had established a marital pattern of disintegrating briefly before picking ourselves up and coming together. She half breathed, half laughed and asked me, "So your husband hasn't checked out, huh?"

Erin's answer didn't fully register until later. Walking down the street the next day, I thought about her words. Her husband had checked out. Not Drew. After we fought, we always came back. Neither of us could get back inside ourselves without resolution. Maybe Erin's boy's self-containment was a devil's bargain for her fractured marriage. But my children had us.

That was when I decided to stop wishing I were a different kind of mother. I stopped wishing I were a different person—a salty mother from New England like my cousins or a mother from Nebraska, where I imagined everyone spoke deliberately. I would stop wanting to be a mother with the kind of squint that made people avert their eyes, forcing them to use their ears. And I would stop replaying and editing conversations so that my sentences were somehow charmingly effective.

I would let Erin's courage surge through me and accept her generous assumption that I was as strong as she was. Like her, I was a warrior mother now—a Valkyrie. Instead of becoming invisible to myself, I could look directly into the eyes of other parents and think: *somewhere, sometime, within the context of your own lives,* **you are me.** An apt cliché: "Everyone has a story." Mine? I looked back at my lone shopping excursions in search of healthy food for my son. Long days. Longer nights. But I had wielded my weapons and fought for my child in those supermarket aisles to the tunes of desolate Muzak.

Chapter 5
FEEL HER BEATING

EDEN COULDN'T HAVE STARRED IN HIS own Lifetime movie. His face didn't hold the pained expressions of a stereotypical sick yet ever-patient child ready for his close-up. In the time of his worst health, when Eden's daytime was an ongoing digestive rumpus and his nighttime was an unrelenting itch, he developed a keen and audible ability to identify exits. As soon as we entered a doctor's office, he would thrust his finger at the door and shrill, "*Dat* way! *Dat* way!" He wanted out, and he let us know it.

Sometimes I wanted to submit to his innocent commands, to turn toward the exit, grab the knob, and pad out before the doctor entered. Though I couldn't tell Eden, I knew exactly where "that way" was. That way held our springy mattress where Eden rolled and bounced and never fell. While he flipped and flew, Drew and I leaned over with smiley, goofy faces. That way was where helicopters soared through the sky, reaching the clouds, and never ever disappeared behind buildings to taunt Eden with an invisible chopping thrum. That way was where his light-up toys never ran out of batteries. It was weeks of freedom from doctors or appointments.

I had been that way often with Dayna, my well child, but I hadn't looked around when she was young and fully appreciated the effortless fortune of her good health. It's said that newborns spend the first week of life in shades of gray. Then come the colors. Eden showed me that every parent travels between this way and that way with his or her children, shifting between the tints of joy and danger, adventure and fear, health and sickness.

When Dayna was just born, I shamed Drew into whispering his way through our dinners while Dayna, deep in her newborn rapid eye movement (REM) sleep, snapped her eyes open, rolled them back, and then fell still again. I breathed the sharp smell of her scalp through my nose like an addict, my pleasure dampened by fear that it would mellow. When she was learning to walk, I hunched and shuffled behind her for hours despite the admonitions: "She won't break, you know."

Though I had taught children of different ages, when Dayna was born, I felt woefully ill prepared to handle a preverbal child, otherwise known as a baby. When she was almost one year old, I enrolled in a child development class run by a child psychologist named Sally. At those classes, Sally dispensed basic advice in a flat, self-confident Midwestern twang. Looking back, her suggestions appear painfully obvious. I didn't need her expertise as much as I needed to hear expertise from an expert to validate common wisdom when I lacked the confidence to carry through on it.

When most of our children were close to two years old, one mother asked Sally about riding the bus. Her daughter was a runner, a zoomer, and a grabber with angelic blond ringlets. The mother began, "Liza gets crazy on the bus. She won't stay in her seat at all."

"How often do you take the bus?" Sally asked as a red-haired boy pushed a fire truck past her feet.

I let myself drift, knowing Dayna had been born with an innate discretion. In public situations, she avoided attention and thanked others unprompted, and she hadn't once run off a curb or out of a gate. "Two going on forty-two!" a sandbox mommy had chirped at me the other day.

" . . . so not all that often." I tuned back in and heard Liza's mother continue. "But it's awful when we do."

"Give her a candy bar. Or a juice box. Kids love those little juice boxes. And put her by the window. Keep her busy," Sally asserted. "These children just need to be doing something."

"Oh," said Liza's mother. And we cocked our heads like chickens. "Oh."

Meanwhile, our toddlers occupied themselves in a modest playroom across the hall, wandering in and out of our room for quick mommy fixes. Dayna was drawn to the plastic washer-dryer set and completed countless loads of laundry while Sally talked toilet training, sleeping, sharing, eating, and general social acclimation. Sally's eyes peered at our semicircle through her wire-rimmed glasses as she recommended that we get "Saturday night sitters to keep that marriage going" and "put 'em to bed early. These kids are tired!"

One of Sally's favorite bits was about food: "Food! You mothers worry too much about what your children eat. Give them a peanut butter sandwich and move on. Move on!"

Despite Sally's old-school wisdom, I found gaps where I might strong-arm a little contemporary A-plus parenting. During the long hours of Dayna's afternoon nap, instead of enjoying my own projects, reading, or writing, I arranged the Fisher-Price Little People into elaborate mise-en-scènes to enhance her postnap floor time. Fearing that plastic was far more toxic than glass, I saved, boiled, and stored Dayna's leftovers in glass baby food jars. In the cold months I never left the house without a steaming washcloth stashed in Tupperware for fear that hand wipes would chill her delicate skin. I let my heart stretch and bend for dangers that weren't there.

Dayna was on winter holiday from preschool when Eden was born. When she returned to school the first day after the New Year, her teachers bent down and gently prodded, "Dayna, are you a big sister now?" Silently, she nodded. What else was there to say?

For the year to follow, Dayna couldn't have known that her brother wasn't feeling well. Four-year-olds don't form coffee klatches around miniature tables to compare notes on siblings. When Eden fussed or puked, Dayna did the fuss-and-puke two-step. She danced around us busily, harmonizing her four-year-old affirmations: "It's okay, Daddy . . . Mommy; it's just what babies do, right? Daddy, Mommy says it's just what babies do."

Dayna had snappy, happy eyes and a thoughtful expression. Her role in the family was that of the persevering sibling, but there were times when I had my doubts about the depth of her cheer. Sometimes, when Eden was raising the roof, Dayna's eyeballs froze in his direction, her face a blank canvas covering the impressions behind it. I knew that face. Drew wore it from time to time. I called it his conference-call face, his eyes unreadable as he tracked voices in his earpiece. Dayna's close-up could be just as inscrutable.

All I knew with certainty was that the drama of Eden's symptoms was unfolding around Dayna. They even shared a bedroom. For example, Eden woke during the night with the frequency of a newborn for several years. Though studies have shown that the kind of eczema-induced sleeplessness he had is fairly typical, the fatigue it caused throughout our family had additional consequences. Cumulative sleep deprivation led to exhaustion, mood swings, and a social breakdown among the members of my family. There are studies on the direct correlations between the severity of sleep disturbance caused by atopic eczema and levels of maternal anxiety.[15] When I thought about Dayna, I wanted to protect her from the feelings of hopelessness, guilt, anger, and depression that can run through parents on red-eyed mornings.

I wanted to believe that Dayna's vibrant preschool playdate circuit and our child-centric apartment replete with toys and an art corner with the ongoing singularly thematic crayon series of smiling girls sporting elephantine bows, along with her randomly timed renditions of the Dreidel Song, were evidence of her happiness. When Drew and I stepped gingerly into the children's room at night, twisting on the dimmer lights to inspect bleeding scratches or measure Benadryl, Dayna lay asymmetrically with her legs in the air or one arm hanging over the side of the bed. I liked to think that she was having sweet dreams. And when Drew and I taped the reminder for Eden's medications on their bedroom door—"Remember Eden's vitamins" punctuated by a happy face—and nightly burst into a round of moronic clapping after Eden swallowed—"*Yaaay. Gre-ee-at job!*"—Dayna surely clapped along with gorgeous sincerity. Surely.

I hope the idyllic Friday afternoons Dayna and I shared during her final year of preschool now float in the clear pools of her subconscious. I looked forward to Friday all week. On Fridays, I took Dayna to her drama class, uninterrupted by Eden's needs. On those Friday afternoons for a period of twelve weeks, I didn't have to wipe spit-up, phone doctors, or record Eden's intake because Dayna had a class in which no strollers were allowed. So every week I left Eden with our part-time sitter or a grandparent and speed walked up to the double-arched wooden doors of Dayna's preschool. I usually arrived just in time to see the doors swing open to reveal cross-legged children sitting in the vestibule. Dayna and I then walked leisurely uptown to her dance school for Dramatic Movement Ages Four to Eight.

We always stopped at the pizzeria on Lexington Avenue, and I was always surprised at the way my hunger crept out of me at the smell of melted cheese and sauce. I would stop at a shop a block farther along for a less messy, wrapped sandwich to take with us. At the school there were long benches underneath the wall of windows where I could sit and watch chubby pink legs thump and twirl beneath pink leotards. Classical music burst in and out of the waiting area as the doors opened for latecomers.

Sandwich balancing easily on my lap, I had a comfortable view of Dayna barefoot, jumping into poses. "Make a shape!" Dayna became a shooting star. "You are lions pouncing and roaring!" Dayna made guttural sounds with abandon, her arms outstretched. I chewed between her spurts of activity. Friday afternoons were safe.

Despite these assurances, throughout Dayna's preschool years I kept watch for signs of discontent. Most mothers keep watch; threats to our children are like ships on the horizon. I wondered if one day Dayna's five-foot FAO Schwarz hippo, Nunga, the Watch Keeper of the Bedroom, would develop a telling outbreak of jungle hives. Or maybe I would come across her squirrel family toppled over in paralyzed surprise after eating poisonous acorns. But no, there were no such symbolic improvisations, no urgent prompt to discuss Eden's illness in greater detail. When I asked Dayna's teachers to keep me informed of any issues, reports home were of an increasingly lively, sharp, and growing girl.

Dayna's head teacher was a large-boned blond, ruddy woman who could hold forty children in her lap at a time, whose hands were forever mixing Play-Doh or paste for multiple projects, and whose body was always covered with a large canvas apron to fend off recriminations for smears and spills.

"Don't worry; if Dayna needs something, she will let you know. They're too young to hold back at this age," she assured me one day at pickup.

I remember thinking how nice it would feel to fold myself into her thick arms, her deep voice enveloping me as I rested for just a few minutes. Instead, I accepted her words as sage and brought Dayna home, with seventeen-month-old Eden strolling in front of us.

As if to underline her teachers' assurances, as Dayna's final year of preschool wound down, she became obsessed with the thematic intricacies of *The Wizard of Oz*. "Why did the flowers make them too sleepy to follow the road?" she asked me repeatedly, never satisfied.

Though Dayna believed in the flying monkeys and stayed taut during their action scenes, she didn't believe my answer that "sometimes flowers can be magical." Her beliefs effectively illustrated the inconsistency of belief.

Dayna began making daily requests for a Dorothy costume and braids. The braids were easy enough to provide, but I couldn't find the time to procure a costume in April. Eventually, one of my alpha-mom friends took pity on my lack of ingenuity and gave me a pair of used ruby red slippers and a blue gingham dress purchased complete with a certificate of authenticity from eBay. So thanks to that MGM spectacle, when Eden was distracting me by, for example, gagging phlegm into his bathwater, my daughter would walk blissfully past the bathroom, hands clasped at her bosom, eyeballs gazing starward, while emoting, "There's no place like home."

When Dayna started kindergarten, Drew and I knew that she might need help dealing with the logistics of her new world, but we didn't predict the emotional divide for her between ages four and five. The October of her kindergarten year, Dayna began to question me about death. This kind of question is never simple, but I had formed some beliefs about death and the afterlife and felt comfortable answering her. I told her that the important part of us lives on, the part that loves. She seemed satisfied, but those first questions were easy compared to the ones that followed: "Which dead animals do we eat?" "Do people eat rabbits?" "Like the bunny at Julia's house?" "Why?" "What about baby animals?" "Do the animals grow up first?" "Why do we eat them at all?"

"Some people but not us." "Sometimes the animals are young, and sometimes they aren't." "People need to eat." I tried to form simple and respectful answers.

On Thanksgiving day, Dayna pushed away her plate of turkey and stage-whispered into my ear, "I don't want to eat dead animals anymore."

Despite her grandparents' offers of more gravy, less gravy, no gravy, ketchup, her eyes glazed with slipping innocence and tears. "I'm sure she doesn't need help," I interrupted the onlookers. "Dee, you can just have some of the mashed potatoes. I know you like potatoes." Dayna had grazed her plates happily and independently since she could put her pincher fingers together, but not so much lately.

"Let's not make this an issue," I told myself as firmly, and repeated that message to Drew later that night, knowing full well that eating was an issue in our home whether we wanted it there or not.

"Well, your house smells like a hamburger. Most of the time," my mother noted a few weeks later. She had dropped by while I was preparing dinner. The days were shortening rapidly, and I opened the kitchen window to let the gamy fumes of frying meat out into the night air. I couldn't make much of a rebuttal since I was at that moment experimenting with one of Ben's suggestions: grass-fed beef. The brand he had suggested was gamy and tough (at least the cuts I could afford), and in truth, my mother was being tactful: our house smelled like a barnyard, not a hamburger.

"It's this meat." I sighed. "It's like chewing gum."

Like many children, Dayna had neatly connected the sustenance on her plate to the source of the sustenance. All at once, her eating changed from a relatively thoughtless act driven by sensory pleasure into an exercise in questions and regard. Her awareness was well timed to a period when I had many more questions than answers about how and what our family should be eating. When it came to Eden's diet, I knew I stood squarely on the side of animal protein. Meat was Eden's safest and most viable food. So what if passing dogs salivated at my stroller bag?

First, I decided that if Dayna needed to pass on dead animals for a while, that was "just fine." She seemed willing to eat other protein sources. Mind you, all the alternative proteins I could come up with (eggs, beans, cheese, nuts, and soy) made me tense because I feared cross-contamination. Reluctantly, I devised food and table rules for Dayna: (1) Almond butter was permitted, but only if Dayna ate it outside our home (her school was peanut-free, and illogically, the smell of peanut butter scared me more than the smell of other nut butters). (2) Soy milk must stay in a covered cup, though she was getting old for those lids. My choice of soy milk over cow's milk was based on her preference and again was somewhat arbitrary in terms of Eden's multiple food allergy safety. (3) Hand rinsing after meals was encouraged in lighthearted yet firm tones. Justifications for new rules made daily appearances. For example, one day I turned suddenly against wrappers, rampaging on her "inappropriate" use of the foil wraps from Hershey's Kisses as craft scrap. At Dayna's tender age, I had amassed a fiefdom of craft scrap, hoarding sticky Now and Later wrappers, bottle caps, and my father's transparent cigar casings. But that was another time altogether.

It seemed to me that Dayna began eating less and less food, not just meat. Despite my efforts to appear both easy breezy and earth mama, grounded about this trend, we both noticed. Dayna was smiling less too.

"Maybe she's not hungry because she's sitting for longer periods in her classroom," I suggested to Drew. "It's winter. Less exercise?"

He set her nearly full plate by the sink, where I was scraping and stacking dishes. "Maybe. Or maybe," he countered, "she's just having her first really picky phase. It's her age?"

Maybe. So we continued with a feigned "I'm not concerned, Dayna will eat when she's hungry" stance for the duration of that winter. Eden's second birthday passed, and Dayna continued to trudge off to kindergarten. In the spring I created my seminal chocolate cake. For a few months, I thought that cake would be Dayna's salvation, too. It felt so good to eat the cake together that I underplayed how little hunger Dayna showed for anything. She had stopped caring whether her food was from the dead animal or vegetable kingdom—the same beans I had been making for a year suddenly looked "like poop," and the edges of her favorite omelet were "too rough." *Let her eat cake? Just cake?*

When the next school year began, it seemed like everything bothered Dayna. She found endless sources of angst: For some reason, she often found the bathroom conducive to self-expression. Brushing her teeth reminded her that her first loose tooth wouldn't fall out despite ongoing wiggling. "I just want it to come out! What can we do?" Stepping into the shower, she informed me of her diminutive status. Dayna was the second smallest girl in the class. "Only Ming Ming is smaller, but everyone *thinks* I'm the smallest!" Dayna's shoulder bones arched like butterfly wings as she shrugged at the injustice of her classmates' misjudgments. New reasons for malaise emerged daily: "Did you know I have gym class tomorrow and I don't like gym class?" I did. "Did you know gym class is always on Wednesday and that's why I don't like Wednesdays?" She questioned me thoroughly, prepared to display distress no matter what my response was.

Ironically, Dayna still enjoyed strong physical health. School notices traveled home in her backpack warning of contagious strep throat and lice, but viruses and bugs mostly kept their distance. Thus, there was no medical justification to see our pediatrician, Ben. So what? So what if I had a child with a small appetite who was a tad cranky from the long school day? So what if I felt like a new character in *Green Eggs and Ham* with one child who "could not" and one child who "would not."

Then again, maybe Ben's outside-the-box medical attention could point me toward some simple solutions. I was still seeing Doctor Reiss. I guessed I could check after Dayna with her as well. So after Ben's thorough and unhurried exam, we left Dayna to play in the outer room while we sequestered ourselves in his inner office.

"She's fine," he assured me. "I would like for her to eat more, but serious intervention can backfire. There is no reason to panic. I would try reading the *Little House on the Prairie* series to encourage her appreciation of homespun cooking and people who lived and fed themselves in tandem with nature." Then he added, "Oh. And do call me if this doesn't get resolved. I have an unusual option."

At my next appointment with Doctor Reiss, I updated her on my predicament. With her predictable blend of perception and practicality, she suggested, "Dayna might be feeling danger in a way she can't verbalize. You can't entirely hide the dangers of food in your home. A short ritual might do the trick. She needs something tangible that will allow her to eat freely. Whatever she is sitting down to, she needs that food to feel sanctified and safe."

Together, Doctor Reiss and I pondered the possibility of mealtime prayers, of simple thanks before our everyday meals, in particular to the animals we consumed for our nourishment. Words might spirit away any remnants of mixed emotions and stringent dietary restrictions. Words might take the obvious jitter out of Drew's eyes when, for example, Dayna saluted us with a party bag filled with Cadbury chocolate-covered peanut butter hearts after a schoolyard Valentine's Day exchange or I had the nerve to buy a new brand of ketchup.

Prayers. Hypothetically I knew something about them. I had attended Hebrew school until my bat mitzvah. But then, like my parents, I saved family prayers for Hanukkah, the Jewish New Year, and Passover. Every spring my father stood at the head of the table holding a silver kiddush cup, chanting blessings and bobbing into his collarbone. We thanked God for the bread and the wine, for candlelight, and for taking us out of slavery thousands of years ago. We did not thank him (or her) for the leftover apple crisp that my brother and I had fought over the night before or for the reupholstered seat cushions we sat on or for my mother's new fax machine in her home office on the other side of the dining room. Our God wasn't interested in those kinds of things.

As I fanned my fingers on the edge of the table, shifting my weight from hip to hip, my breath would rise and fall with my father's singsong Hebrew. He was someone else then, and for those few moments I was lost. It was easy to determine that to pray was to lose oneself. I didn't want to go wherever my father already was. So I was a fake, mumbling along with him.

Drew's mother may have cooked up a few holiday meals for her children, but he can't really remember. They did not pray together. Drew's maternal grandfather emigrated from Jerusalem with the conviction that he and his family must embrace America and all that it stood for, not old-world Jewish values. He brought his daughter up accordingly. One of Drew's mostly fondly remembered childhood dinners was his grandparents' weekly visit. First they would watch the *CBS Evening News* in his mother's bedroom. Then his grandfather would fry up his specialty of breaded flounder fillets. While they sat around the dining room table, his grandfather carefully explained that week's current events to his grandsons. It was a lovely ritual if you ask me.

When Drew and I met, religion wasn't very important to either of us. Anyway, we were familial Jews, which meant our parents wouldn't worry. As a couple, we had opted to celebrate the Jewish holidays. Most of them, at least. And of course we amped up our routines after we had Dayna. We joined a temple that we never attended outside the children's services and programs, and at the time Doctor Reiss made her suggestion to me about establishing gratitude at the table, we didn't have daily observances.

The night after meeting with Doctor Reiss, I made chicken soup from scratch, a dish Dayna had preapproved despite her quasi-vegetarianism. Eden was dining on hot dog soup, a dish designed by his feeding therapist. The recipe was built around thinly sliced Applegate Farm turkey dogs. (Applegate Farm had a heartwarming pledge on its website to "never hide any known allergen behind this label ['natural flavorings'].") After you cook the hot dogs, you stir them into a bowl of Beech-Nut brand carrot puree. Last, add a small portion of cooked corn and stir with confidence. Now everyone can have soup.

I brought three bowls to the table. But when I sat down at our white Formica table, I became overeager, crashing in before Dayna had picked up her spoon, "Dayna, let's say thank you for this yummy soup we're eating, okay? Let's see. Let's see. . . . Thank you, carrots, for growing so sweet and letting someone pick you, and thank you, chicken, for, um, being part of our soup too because, uh, you make it taste even better than it would, uh, without you there, and I'm just so *glad* we have our dinner to eat tonight."

"Okay. But Mommy, what about the rice?" she asked, ever thorough. "There's rice in the soup too."

"Well, we don't have to go through everything, but we can if you want . . . it's just . . . the idea . . . uhh . . . what do you think we should say about the rice?" Two minutes into this venture and my awkwardness had cloaked any audible spirituality. I was used to praying in another language, and now I was trying to pray with everyday words. They were phone call words, bossy words, laughing and lying words. I was rearranging my words to sound like more than what they were, as if I could make them holy. I could not. I didn't believe in them or in myself.

"Anyway, I don't like chicken soup when it has rice," Dayna announced.

"So just have the broth and the chicken," I suggested, spooning Eden's soup into his open mouth. He was already clamoring for his bowl.

"But the chicken has weird things coming off it. *Strings.* Can I leave it and just have the broth?" Once she had maligned my soup with that word—*strings*—the gastronomical equivalent of *blobs* and my secret word for those icky opaque undercooked parts of scrambled eggs, I knew I had failed.

"Okay, Dee, okay . . ." I wallowed away, mentally and physically, into a mist of guilt.

I was the picky one in a family of fearless eaters. I was pick-pickity queen of the pickers, the only member of my family to smother veal cutlets in ketchup and the only one who reeled upon sighting my father's caraway-seeded cole slaw. "But they look like bugs!" I objected shamelessly. My repulsion was powerful and commanding. Deep within, I teetered under the weight of those simple memories and a more complex question: If Dayna, at her age, could not grasp the ungodly truth that certain foods were the equivalent of keeping a loaded gun in our home, could she nevertheless sense the random nature of Eden's problem? Did she ask herself why her brother and not her? Had food become associated with danger, and was she trying to protect herself from it?

And what was the seismic alternative? Easy. I was projecting. There was an embarrassing possibility there, an oopsee-doopsee silly mommy likelihood that Dayna was just having a hard year (age and stage). But I couldn't gauge the truth because of our recent family history: Drew and I had just begun to process the implications of Eden's condition, and as with her stubborn tooth, Dayna was stuck within our reality. Some things were better. My fifteen minutes of fame as a chocolate cake baker had given me the confidence to bake and cook in odd but safe ways. We were all eating more, and our food even tasted better. Eden was beginning to heal too. His body was less volatile. Dayna might need more time to catch up.

The night we tried to pray I had a dream. Dayna hid spaghetti in her pants pockets and refused to take the pants off. Instead she stood defiantly in front of me, hips jutted, the wet red strands dripping down her long lean thighs.

"Hanukkah," I promised myself aloud the next morning. That seemed a fitting deadline. "I'll decide what to do after Hanukkah." The winter holidays were approaching, and Dayna looked forward to Hanukkah every year. Maybe a child-centered holiday replete with presents and eggless potato pancakes would recharge her.

But Hanukkah came and went. We chuckled over Eden's confusion as he commanded us to "Blow! Blow!" as soon as we lit our menorah, and Dayna smirked along. But that was all. It was an otherwise uneventful time in their lives. Although it was a challenge to keep two children busy in an apartment during the winter, Dayna was the more self-contained child. She was learning to read books with long chapters, albeit reluctantly since she loved hearing stories aloud. We tried to encourage her new skill by taking the kids on regular trips to the library. When we didn't have any particular excursions planned or I couldn't secure playdates, Dayna gravitated toward a small well-worn wooden table in the corner of the dining room. She was a master craftsman, and Eden, always eager to shadow her behavior, gripped his crayons and drew alongside her.

That year we bought the children a toy that involved spin art, the classic pastime in which children squeeze paint into a spinning plastic disk and then spin the disk as it shoots out droplets of rainbow patterns onto paper. I stood over Dayna and Eden or crouched by their table, and they alternately hovered and squeezed. They looked on with the kind of awe I tended not to appreciate until after the fact. I did tape almost all their work on the walls, and I did remember to continue to express culinary thanks and gratitude until well after the New Year. But I didn't see any visible changes in Dayna's subdued mood or appetite.

It was March and we were up to *By the Shores of Silver Lake* when I decided to take up Ben on his ambiguous option. He returned my daytime call at nearly nine o'clock that night, apologizing for the late hour. "I just didn't want to keep you waiting," he explained. That was *so* Ben.

"I'm just glad we can talk," I answered. "Let me get Drew to pick up the other phone." Drew picked up the other handheld in the bedroom, and we lay on our bed side by side.

"I've been thinking about Dayna, and the option I want to offer has brought several of my patients and friends success. But it's unusual." After a slight pause Ben went on: "I would have you call a distance healer named William Miller."

Our heads whipped toward each other, Drew's eyebrows raised, mine furrowed. With those expressions frozen in place, we listened while Ben told four detailed anecdotes about a man from Santa Fe, New Mexico, who could heal people over the phone. He worked with their "energy" through the phone. After seeing his success with several clients with physical and emotional issues, Ben tested William Miller personally. He simply asked the healer, "How do *I* look?" "I didn't tell him anything else, because I wanted to know whether he was building on information he already knew," Ben confided.

We responded with mumbling and fresh head gyrations.

William Miller had reported that Ben was quite fit and happy but plagued by lower back stiffness, which could be rectified easily by daily stretching.

"Absolutely true," Ben affirmed. "It's my only health issue, and he found it! I never mentioned it."

After we thanked Ben and hung up, Drew and I turned to each other, each leaning on an elbow. "Okay."

"Okay."

"Can we do this?" we asked each other. What we meant was "Can *we* do this?" Were we trying to find a magic Dayna fix with a wave of a shaman stick? For God's sake, we lived in a high-rise building in New York City. Could energy vibes sneak past the front door, past the service people, and up the elevator?

It got late. Finally, Drew sank his head into his pillow, yawned, and pointed out, "It's not like he can make it worse. Even if he's a fake, he's never going to see or touch Dayna."

"Why not? We'd do it for Eden if Ben had said that this, um, energy person cures allergies. Wouldn't we?" We agreed.

With the lights out and Drew breathing rhythmically, I hugged my pillow, remembering something that used to make Dayna very happy. It was her heartbeat. When she first discovered her heartbeat, it impressed her no end. "Feel my beating," she used to request, smiling broadly several times a day, pulling my hand to her ribs. "Can you feel it?"

Then I thought about Eden: his heart and his hardwired body. Eden had all those allergic antibodies perched on his intestinal walls, nostrils, and lungs, those hateful antibodies that lay there waiting, poised to attack. Just one protein molecule, an invisible speck of egg white in a pan, could beckon Eden's body to release those troublemakers, histamines. They in turn would dilate his blood vessels, release mucus, and ravage his body in their frenzied activity.

Eden needed me to control those reactions if one should begin, and he needed me to control our lives in certain ways. Although I couldn't control Dayna's emotions, I desperately wanted to make her feel safe. I wanted to adopt Drew's "whatever it takes" until she let me know when to stop. Maybe I had to take a different kind of risk for this energy healer to help me do that. Maybe I had to take a risk, suspend my disbelief, shelve my logic and learning just when I had assumed that they were to be intractable tenets of my family's life together.

About two weeks later on the night of our appointment with William Miller, it was cold but not cold enough to put off the Saint Patrick's revelers. I heard bar hoppers piping in from our open kitchen window: "Whooo! Wa-hoo! Yeah!"

My cryptic yellow Post-it on our refrigerator read "6:00 pm W. M." As if more detail might have caused random interrogations about my spiritual convictions as evidenced by telltale Post-its. It was almost six o'clock. Drew sat cross-legged on the floor with Eden, constructing a LEGO oven to bake his plastic bread slices. Dayna was in front of the small television in our bedroom watching *Cyberchase*, a show in which cyberchildren flying in cybercrafts fight an evil villain by using their mathematical skills. It felt like a good thematic choice for the evening ahead.

When William and I spoke to make the appointment, his smooth, deep voice steadied my chirpy sounds. "Uhh . . . so . . . ? Ben thought you might be able to help us."

"Please call me William, not Mr. Miller," he answered, and that made me feel even sillier.

William began by describing his résumé: a large tossed salad of alternative healing methods, including astrological charting, Ayurveda-based nutrition, and herbal medicine. However, he didn't specify which school of thought had enabled him to heal across the time zones. And he told me he had children. Important.

William asked for the date, location, and time of Dayna's birth; informed me that he would do some "preparations"; and set up a telephone appointment. If Dayna didn't want to speak to him, that was fine. She just needed to be in the same room as me.

"Would it be okay if she's watching TV?" I asked with immediate regret. *TV? So uncool.*

But he said simply, "It's fine. No problem."

When the phone rang that Friday night, I took it into the bedroom, where Dayna was lying on our queen-size bed, fresh from a shower. Her chestnut-brown hair wet the collar of her T-shirt and the pillows propped behind her. William asked me a few more questions about Dayna: her food preferences, her favorite activities, and her health. Then he stopped talking, and all I could hear was mumbling and breathing.

I heard paper sliding and fluttering, something that could have been chanting or not, words that could have been English or not, and after a while I got drowsy. My gaze shifted between *Cyberchase* and our white bedroom wall. The edges of our framed wedding photo softened as my eyes lost focus. For a long time nothing seemed to be happening. "Are you sure you don't want me to turn the TV off?"

"No, no, she is cooperating in her own quiet way," he assured me. "Now I'm going to work a little inside her."

His breathing noises slowed, and just as I began to free-float into self-mockery, Dayna, who had been immobile since the opening bars of the *Cyberchase* theme song, touched her mouth. She gently rubbed her fingertips against her lips with one hand. After about two minutes of rubbing, she put her hand down and, as delicately as a woman who doesn't want to smear her lipstick, smacked her lips and swallowed. I hadn't moved my eyes from her face.

She turned to me and whispered, "'Excuse me, but I'm really, really thirsty." With William's permission (he was still going, as it were), I got up and brought her a cup of water from our bathroom, which she took without looking at me, eyes back on the television screen.

Shortly afterward, William told me he was finished. We had a discussion about "stoking" Dayna's digestive fires with some spicy foods and teas. He suggested that I use more spices in her food and consider making her homemade lemonade. Finally, he asked me if I ever tried saying mantras or prayers with Dayna. "Yup. Doesn't work. We can't really pray over food." As if I hadn't made my position clear, I added, "Tried it a lot."

"Well," he said, and paused, "you can still be glad about food, glad that it's there to nourish you. You can let her know when you feel that way." The timbre of his voice could not have been kinder.

"I will think about that." What I meant was, *Since I trusted in you to adjust my daughter's psychic energy, you might have rightfully assumed that I'm spiritual enough to muster gratitude about nourishment, so I don't want to disappoint you at this moment.*

"Nothing will happen for three days," he predicted. "Let's follow up in a week so I can hear about her."

And then we were done.

Later that night, Drew and I couldn't choose dinner. "Chicken Parm?" he asked, shuffling our stack of paper menus.

"Too heavy." I held my hand out for the stack.

A few minutes later we mashed two cans of tuna fish and brought a sleeve of Carr's crackers to the table. When we finished eating, Drew cleared around me while I wrote William Miller a check. Peeling the stamp off, I imagined the adobe-walled kitchen where he would open the envelope, the smells of his chipotle-seasoned vegetarian repasts, the New Mexican late day sun slanting into his window.

For a moment I wanted to grab Drew's wrist and tell him that without delay we must pack up our essentials, stuff duffels into the car, and drive, fly, or cyberport ourselves to a place where the color of earth would be just outside our door. Was this entire exercise a sign, a signal to reshape our lives once again? Was it time to give Dayna her turn?

Three days later, my brother Charlie drove into the city for the day with my two-year-old nephew Sam. Temperatures had risen, but the sun was still being coy. Generally there isn't much to do outdoors in Manhattan in March, but I had a firm fresh-air policy: If there wasn't water on the ground or coming out of the sky, we played outside for as long as we could stand it. I was grateful that Charlie and Sam were there that morning to liven up the playground.

After about an hour of tag and sliding and shrugging our shoulders and mumbling "Whoof!" we surrendered to lunch. Walking west out of the park, Drew split off with Eden at Second Avenue as planned while my brother and I continued downtown in search of a restaurant with a free booth.

"We need to close Sam in," Charlie asserted, snuffing Sam's nose with tissue. "He'll stand up and stay up on a freestanding chair. Trust me."

After Charlie had stuck his head into at least four restaurants, we compromised on a questionable joint called the Mustang Grill, popular for its margarita-fueled happy hours. The Southwest was the theme of our week, I guessed, sliding into a booth surrounded by peeling amber walls with matching peeling cactus decals. Dayna fretted over the menu, finally requesting French fries and French toast from the waiter despite my insistence that "that might not be such a good combination, honey." I stroked her arm while we waited for our food.

Sure enough, four bites into the greasy Cajun-dusted fries and deep-fried French toast, Dayna turned to me, wet pain washing her eyes. "I don't feel good at all; my loose tooth hurts so much, like my stomach."

Sensing there was more of something to come, I excused both of us to gallop the three blocks home on a day that was already bleak with dark afternoon clouds. As we approached our front door, Dayna repeated for the tenth time, "I *really* don't feel good. Not at all. *Oh, Mom.*"

Then she leaned into my chest and wept. It was a cloudburst. I felt her tears pooling in a tangled mat of hair. It smelled like damp French fries. Silently I waited, my chin tucked into her head. She hadn't cried like that in a long time. Suddenly Dayna's head popped up like a deer, so close that the edges of her face were fuzzy. All I could see was her open red mouth. And in the middle of her mouth, on her tongue, there was a small white square. I pulled it off before she could swallow.

"Your tooth!" Now tearless, holding hands, we went into the bathroom to rinse her mouth.

After we washed and solemnly examined the tooth, Dayna's eyes lit up. "I feel so much better now. I think I just want to lie down."

"Of course." I ushered her to our faded couch, covered her with a white throw, and lay next to her until she fell asleep. I rose over her. There was a sheen of sweat on her hairline. Dayna never lay down during the day unless she was very sick. I scurried into the kitchen to whisper my theories to Drew. He had kept himself at the periphery since Dayna and I had walked in.

"I think she just had a healing crisis. I've read about this thing where, like, things get so bad and then come together, but I think the tooth is like a sign of purging or something. What do you think?" I whispered fast, ignoring Eden, who was at our feet, removing all the pots from a kitchen cabinet.

"Something's going on," he said. At that moment, I was frustrated with Drew's broad-stroke analysis when I thought I had procured a tangible explanation. But in the end it didn't really matter what we believed or what really happened. We had done something to help our other child when she needed it. The very thought was salve for years to come.

Dayna dozed until her bath time, and when she woke, her lips parted in a slight Alfred E. Newman grin as she asked for black beans and maybe a fried egg. I didn't dare disagree, but I prepared the food apprehensively, wishing she had asked instead for plain toast and jelly. But after finishing the first plateful, she asked for more and then finished the second portion. *Hmm.* I ate my dinner by her side. Hmm.

The next night at dinner, Dayna looked at her pasta and asked, "Can I mix some lettuce in? I want something green and crunchy in it." A week later she said, "Remember how you used to make me cheese and pickle sandwiches for lunch?" I remembered. "I want sandwiches again. Sometimes. And cinnamon apples."

Although she didn't request any meat for months to come, Dayna began to eat more and then more until she returned to us with her bad days and better days, her eyes rounded over drippy pizza, her oatmeal bowl scraped clean, her smiles and her stone-still listening face, her old and then new habits, all of her familiar. When Dayna was eleven years old, the Food Allergy and Anaphylaxis Network published a monthly newsletter that featured a cover article on the connection between food allergies and disordered eating among children. Although the article was focused on children with food allergies, not their siblings, it asserted that "disordered eating" as opposed to "eating disorders" is "much more common among individuals with food allergies . . ." Not surprising. I will never know if the timing and circumstances of Dayna's dead animals repulsion related to Eden's food allergies. In fact, by the time that newsletter arrived, Eden's seven-year-old collarbone showed and his ribs visibly flexed. My children were, and still are, thin. And Eden is very choosy about meat, preferring as little as possible. But now I'm certain that Dayna is well nourished by her place in our family and so by her food. And when there was food strife, when Eden was suffering, Dayna found a way to carve a leading role for herself.

Now she cheerleads. When Eden is worried about an upcoming event at which his food might suffer by comparison, Dayna excels in pushing back against his anxiety. For example, last spring there was a brief period when Eden indulged in an uncharacteristic amount of Sturm und Drang regarding his food restrictions. And one day in May, after I'd walked the children home from school and they'd cozied up to our dining room table for snacks and homework, Eden popped his head up and asked, "Guess what?" As usual, he paused for the "What?" yet something in his voice made me wish I didn't have to ask.

"Our class is running the make-your-own-cupcake booth at the spring fair!" he reported, and then pressed his lips tightly. He looked down, breathed in.

Dayna was sitting next to him while I sat on the other side, sorting mail and then reflexively drumming up a list of cupcake options at nanosecond speed. She and Eden listened intently while I fell back on my can-do routine: "Nooo problem, Eden! I'll bake our safe cupcakes, and you know what we can do? We'll bring a bottle of that chocolate syrup you love and our chocolate chips and you can help the other kids with allergies make their own cupcakes too!"

I continued more along the vein of Tyra Banks telling her Next Top Models to "rock those cupcakes! Rock 'em now, people!" than that of a mother who truly believed in what she was saying. These would be the same cupcakes plus the same go-to topping we had used for all impromptu and allergically baffling dessert situations during the last four years. Would that be anywhere near as exciting as choosing a cupcake from hundreds in order to spackle on mounds of Duncan Hines frosting, heap on M&M's, and bury the entirety in sprinkles?

Then Dayna broke in. "Wait a minute, Eden. I swear I'm not just saying this." As she spoke, she raised her palm forward in a hybrid pledge of childhood guarantee that her next words would be nothing but the truth.

Leaning forward over her laptop, she waited until his gaze moved upward from our khaki tablecloth and into hers. Then she said, "Wait. That *seriously* sounds so much better than those cupcakes they always sell that I would so much rather eat that. Wait. You are seriously lucky. I *wish* I could buy one of them at the fair, but you should probably save them for the other kids with allergies."

Why wouldn't Eden believe her every word? She was the authority on the politics and preferences of grade school children, and we all knew it. Her unique validation permitted the conversation to move on to possible color options at the upcoming hair-painting booth. And several minutes later, after they had wound down, their faces bent toward worksheets, I interrupted: "Are you done with those plates?"

Their heads lifted in tandem and their eyes went straight to me, giving me the same look, the kind of look that said, "And you are *who* . . . ?"

Those looks were my proof that I didn't have a well or a sick child. I had children who had different needs at different times. In Dayna's case, much like her brother, she had experienced a negative reaction to something whose source we could only guess at. Whatever it was, she could not control it. I can't explain how William Miller helped Dayna, but engaging with him gave us the strength to continue our journey with all its unexpected chances and rewards.

Chapter 6

MEDICINE MOM

ONE MID-FEBRUARY MORNING YEARS AGO, I was teaching a middle-school English class when a fishy odor wafted into my classroom. Pregnant with Dayna that year, I spent September to December excusing myself during classes to nearly retch in the girls' bathroom. Leaning my head against the cool stalls, I wished for many things. Sometimes I wished I had chosen to work in a corporate environment where teenagers weren't allowed to roam like wolfhounds, sniffing me out. Sometimes I wished I hadn't eaten breakfast in my puppy dog optimism that this time scrambled eggs would be just the thing. I always wanted to empty my stomach, but as I later confirmed when carrying Eden, my pregnancy wiring cut short at vomiting and left me in perpetual nausea.

That year I had a very allergic student named Alex. He was often absent, and it affected his already poor academic organization. During our fall parent-teacher conference, Alex's parents described his allergies and asthma as well as the resulting infections and colds. It seemed ironic to me that Alex was allergic to innumerable icons of childhood, including peanut butter and jelly sandwiches, puppies, and stuffed animals. How odd, I thought.

The day of the fish odor, Alex's class was scheduled just before lunch. The school building was so narrowly vertical that it gave the cafeteria fumes efficient passage up into my classroom. For two periods, students had burst through my door and thumped into their desks. "Ewww, that's foul! It really is! No way am I eating lunch today!"

More than halfway through Alex's class, the smell intensified. It seemed those fish were taunting us, curling their oily charred edges in our direction. When Alex raised his hand, a student named Justine was reading aloud. Bad timing. I had just caught her fiddling with what looked like a fuzzy hybrid mouse-snake attached to a key chain. So when Alex signaled me, I returned my wait-a-minute signal.

Instead Alex scraped his chair back. "I'm sorry, but I have to go to the nurse! I have to. I'm allergic to fish!"

Mutters from the back row, "Yeah, *right*."

I was losing time. I wanted to present essay topics by the next week. There was shuffling, fuzzy movement in my periphery.

"No, really!" Alex objected, though I hadn't opened my mouth. "I feel like I can't breathe. I need my medicine!"

Then he was in front of my desk, and I pulled out the permission pad from the drawer. "Okay, but wait for a slip." I kept my eyes on him as I bent over it to write.

"I *need* my medicine!"

His medicine. I don't know how I knew, but I did. I retracted. "No. Don't. Don't wait. Go! Go get it."

He was gone.

Alex got his medicine. After class I checked on him, and he was fine, so I didn't give it much thought until fourteen years later, when I read that cooking is a clinically proven means of releasing airborne allergens. Fourteen years later I carried Eden through the double doors of a hospital emergency room. Our second time. That second time wasn't about food. It was about airborne allergens.

Eden wasn't a silent bloated baby then like the previous time, but he was still in my arms, his heart hammering into my shoulder. He was calm. He repeated, "Hospital?" his breath raspy in my ear. He had heard me throw the word into the air for Drew to catch just as I was catapulting us out the door. "Hospital?" Eden could have been saying "Snail?" or "Mailbox?" It was another new word.

"Yes, hospital," I answered. "To help you feel better. That's all." Spring had been making promises all day, whispering about heat and colors. And the air was still thick, already dark as the double glass doors hummed open. Then we stood in front of a clerk behind a glass entryway, the first outpost.

"Was he born here?" she asked. He was, and that meant no more questions after laboring through the spelling of our last name.

"That's W-e-i."

"His doctor called you in. You can go right there." She pointed at the next set of doors. "And happy Mother's Day," she added, deadpan, an emergency room Hallmark card.

Her words didn't sink in because within a minute I was trying to grasp the next phrase: "He's in respiratory distress." The clerk told me to carry Eden to a heavy wooden desk where a nurse put a small clamp on his finger. The clamp sounded quickly, "Beep! Beep! Beep!" The nurse said, "Very high. He's in respiratory distress."

After the finger clamp, the nurse came with me as I carried Eden to a group treatment room. Nick at Nite flashed across the television screen. Another nurse extended a cupped oxygen mask. She was the first of many who would repeat, "Yeah. Respiratory distress."

With Eden on my lap, my hand sweated onto the plastic of the mask. While we waited for a doctor, Eden stared into each smudged corner of the room's entrance. He looked quite normal now. His cheeks were rounded and slightly pink. He didn't look like a little boy who had, seconds before, been in respiratory distress. But why would I trust what I saw?

For a month, Eden had snuffled, sniffed, and blinked rapidly along with a veritable chorus line of Manhattanites. There were record high pollen counts that spring. I had seen pedestrians lurching off curbs in violent sneezes. But maybe none of that would have mattered, I guessed, if we hadn't rented the house. Drew thought the house would be good for us.

Over the previous nine months, finally, we had begun to walk the same line as a family. For the first time since Eden's birth, we had built up days and even weeks of normal. There were weeks of playing, working, and at least some resting. I began to write about Eden to make sense of our lives and what was happening. Drew had helped me select a sturdy silver laptop and a black case.

We pulled together a budget for an off-season rental house on Long Island. Dayna started first grade. Over those months, our weekends outside the city became the fulcrum of our weeks. Eden and Dayna pedaled new bicycles with training wheels. Drew and I sniffed at the exhaust-free air with self-congratulations. There was an electric teakettle. There were pilled couch pillows, untamed shrubs, and snowmen that valiantly withstood our week's absence between the building and the melting. We kept a box of Band-Aids on the coffee table. One Saturday in March when the ice over the pool cover thawed into a giant puddle, two misguided ducks adopted our yard, and the children stood at a safe distance, tearing and tossing chunks of Eden's homemade bread. That brown-shingled house was our Walden Pond, marking a rich late winter and spring.

Back in the city, Central Park flaunted its blossoms. Our final weekend approached, and that Saturday Eden woke up coughing. Just here and there. The next morning, Mother's Day, his cough deepened into short, infrequent barks. Circling a sponge inside a plastic cereal bowl, I wondered whether to call our pediatrician or allergist the next morning. *Another virus?*

We drove home, and in the late afternoon, in his bath, Eden began squeaking long high notes out of his open mouth, his face jerking toward the water with each gasp. I lifted him and wrapped him in his striped towel. He spared his wet flesh but sprayed my back and then my front with vomit.

"Need water! Water!" Eden demanded. Then he began panting, his ribs pushing out and drawing in.

"Call Doctor Anderson," I said to Drew. "I think we have to go to the hospital. Call her. I'm going. I'm going to the hospital. Call her."

Now a doctor approached with a white plastic medicine cup. Compliantly, Eden swallowed the contents while the doctor explained, "He won't talk much now. They conserve their breath." He added that Eden would need more steroids along with a cocktail of bronchial medicine and oxygen in ongoing sequences for eight hours or possibly longer. Maybe we would still be there tomorrow. Or maybe we wouldn't. Maybe they would find us a room. Or maybe they couldn't. Things were tight in pediatrics. The doctor would be back soon.

I looked around. To our right, a pair of twins played Game Boy. The boys looked anywhere between seven and ten years old. One of them wore a mask strapped around his buzzed black hair, so his thumbs were free to work the game as he blinked and shifted. On the other side of the room, piles of books, card games, and action figures plus a bulging orange canvas bag encircled another boy. He was pale, pencil-necked. His mother, sitting next to the cargo, shared his pallid glow. Without their earthly baggage anchoring them to stuffed vinyl chairs, they could have been ghosts.

Then Eden's back relaxed against me. I thought maybe it was a sign of relief, of oxygen pumping into his lungs. Easy air. My shirt had dried into a stiff yeasty sheath. The television hollered into the glaring spaces, the remaining air dim where the fluorescent lighting couldn't reach. All the children breathed in and out in soft, breezy synchronization, their faces all masks and eyes.

I couldn't look anymore, but there was nowhere good to go mentally. How hadn't I known that Eden was having asthma? *Mom has asthma.* I used to hear her in the mornings, the successive deep, wet coughs quieted by her first sips of black coffee. *But her ribs never pumped like that; I never heard her wheeze.* Just then the pale boy distracted me by rustling a bag of Cheese Nips out of his stash. *Cheese Nips?* How could I have forgotten? Our rations—two diapers, one pair of Bob the Builder red piped underpants, hand wipes, my cell phone, and a half-filled plastic cup of flavored, enriched Rice Dream rice milk. How old was it? The two forgotten Peppermint Patties yesterday were pliable and oozing in my jacket pocket. There were two vending machines in the hallway leading to the room, and of course Mount Sinai's hospital staff surely fed hundreds of patients and employees every day. But the Cheese Nips brought me back to Eden's other reality. *Will you even get hungry?* I stroked Eden's hair. Food, hunger; even in a hospital they were so complicated. Now it seemed that breathing was going to be complicated too.

For Eden it was a twenty-four-hour medical marathon, inhaling cocktails of bronchial dilators, saline, and oxygen. Drew and I swapped off, overlapped. In the middle of the night, we left Dayna with Drew's mother and slept on chairs in an exam room–cum–ad hoc sleep room for Eden. (Pediatrics was indeed tight that weekend.) During our final few hours, as we waited to sign out, we were left to roam the short hallways. Eden, pumped on medication and exhaustion, jazzed ahead of us, singing the chorus of his favorite song (thanks to Dayna): "Follow the yellow brick road, follow, follow . . ." The memory still takes my breath away.

When we returned from the hospital, it seemed that a home decorating fairy had performed a twenty-four-hour renovation on our apartment. When I walked in the front door, our windows sparkled and the crimson paint on the dining room walls appeared richer, redder. I breathed in the clean aroma of Murphy soap and then placed my backpack on the front bench. It was heavy with asthma medication and hospital literature. There was a bottle of liquid steroid; two asthma inhalers; an asthma spacer, which is a short wide tube used for sucking in the inhaled medication; a prescription for a nebulizer, a machine that vaporizes asthma medication into the mouth; and a packet of liquid vials containing a bronchodilator. We were home.

The next day Eden and I returned to the hospital for a follow-up with Doctor Anderson, during which I received another prescription for a medication called Singulair (montelukast sodium.) Eden's coughing and wheezing had stopped, but he was to continue to take oral and inhaled medication for about a week and then Singulair, as a daily medication, after that. When a child with Eden's allergic history has his or her first bout of asthma, there is statistical evidence that it won't be the last. A 2008 study published in the *Journal of Allergy and Clinical Immunology* stated, "Eczema within the first two years of life was clearly associated with an increased risk of childhood asthma in boys but not in girls."[16] The same journal published this fact: 63 percent of babies with severe eczema developed asthma by age eight as opposed to 8 percent of all babies.[17] According to the Centers for Disease Control and Prevention (CDC), in 2007, 29 percent of children with food allergies also had asthma.[18] According to a National Institutes of Health (NIH)–funded study published in the October issue of the *Journal of Allergy and Clinical Immunology*, people with food allergies were nearly seven times more likely than those without them to require ER treatment for their asthma in the 12 months leading up to the study and four times more likely to have asthma.[19] I learned that this efficient progression is commonly called the atopic march or the atopic cascade. The odds weren't with Eden. In medicine, these terms are used to describe individuals who have allergic tendencies.

It was the perfect trifecta of allergies: Eden had anaphylactic food allergies, atopic dermatitis, and asthma. His triggers included various foods, environmental allergens and viruses, and dander, all of which can be the starting points for many allergic equations. In the hospital, we learned that Eden had allergic and viral asthma. Both of those conditions sounded like what they were: Allergic asthma meant that Eden's lungs would inflame when he was exposed to an allergen. In his case, it was probably seasonal pollen that had triggered his first asthma attack, the growth of springtime grass and plants. Viral-induced asthma meant that when Eden caught a virus (a common cold or flu, for example), his lungs had an asthmatic reaction to the virus. Why? We call viruses bugs, but they are really a combination of genes and protein. The way Doctor Anderson explained the problem to me was his IgE antibodies could react to a common cold the same as his other allergens. In fact, Eden often broke out in a small patch of hives when he had a head cold. His earlier tendency to have randomly timed hives now didn't seem so random. In retrospect, my student Alex and his frequent absences made perfect sense. For some individuals, the line between viral symptoms and allergic symptoms is difficult to decipher.

Allergic individuals also have new allergic reactions when they experience new situations and environments. In the years to follow, Eden would sleep in a basement guest room and wake up with a sharp wheeze (mold allergy). He would handle a lacquered snake purchased in Chinatown and develop a hand rash (a chemical allergy, we will guess). And after Eden's first horseback ride we were pretty sure he wouldn't ask for another (horse dander).

Why Eden?

Eden was conceived during a time when environmental researchers were addressing this question: Are we becoming more allergic to the world around us? Since our last day in the weekend house had neatly coincided with Eden's first asthma attack, Drew and I figured the countrified environment was to blame and Eden could count on urban relief. But Eden was conceived at the brink of some telling research regarding global warming, allergies, and city dwellers.

Back in March 2002, Drew and I drove to Long Island for a weekend getaway at a beach resort called Gurney's Inn. Though it once had been considered a luxury spa, the painted walls were faded and the moldings around the famed indoor saltwater pool were cracked and leaking. We didn't mind. We were thrilled to have a weekend to ourselves while my father and his wife stayed with Dayna. We were free to walk the shoreline, free to have a fairly awkward but effective couples massage in the spa, and free to make another child. That same spring researchers working on behalf of the U.S. Department of Agriculture planted something else: a lot of weeds.

The lead researcher, Lewis Ziska, wanted to see how increased carbon dioxide emissions might affect the future of the planet's trees and plants. He suspected that the world was making more allergens. After planting weeds in three sites—an organic farm in western Maryland, a park in a Baltimore suburb, and another park by the city's inner harbor—Ziska waited for results over the next five growing seasons.

The two warmer and more carbon dioxide–enriched sites—the suburbs and the inner harbor—grew larger weeds, but what researchers didn't expect was that the weeds at the urban site would grow a full 10 percent larger. And those weeds produced 60 percent more pollen. The researchers also found that the allergy-causing proteins in each pollen grain were more potent, and with spring often arriving earlier every year, those supersized pollens were also in the air for more days, exacerbating conditions such as hay fever, asthma, and even eczema. Like so many other pieces of Eden's allergy puzzle, the story of Lewis Ziska's research and finding was published two years after Eden's first asthma attack, in June 29, 2008, in the *New York Times Magazine*.[20]

The same uneasy relationship between pollen and industrialization can be found in Japan. In response to an enormous demand for housing and timber after World War II, the Japanese government planted forests of cedar trees, only to let them grow largely untended as they multiplied more quickly than they could be harvested. Currently, it's thought that up to twenty million Japanese (16 percent of the population) have seasonal cedar allergies, especially in cities such as Tokyo.[21] But during our weekend getaway years ago, why would I have given any thought to weeds and the toll of global emissions on worldwide pollen counts? Drew and I were busy. In our plush carpeted hotel room we kept the windows open to the ocean wind and let it wash over us. Glorious.

Eden, in contrast, wasn't feeling at all glorious in the aftermath of his hospital stay. It was late spring, and there was no escaping the pollen. Plus, he was having nightmares. Bad ones. At least once or twice a night we were jolted awake by his sweaty shouts. Come morning, when we asked him about his dreams and screams, Eden replied blankly, "I don't remember," eyelashes batting just once. One night he got out of bed and stood in the middle of the room after a long yell. Those episodes weren't anything like his past awakenings. Those were babyish cries to be held and, later, coherent requests for water or kisses.

I asked Doctor Reiss, "Maybe he's a little traumatized from going to the hospital?" assuming she would know.

"Likely. Very likely. It should pass."

It took a few more weeks to consider the influence of Eden's new medication, Singulair. I wouldn't have questioned Singulair if I hadn't run out of it. It took two days to get Eden's prescription refilled, then I forgot to give it to him for a few *more* days, and then I realized that he had stopped having nightmares. And then I gave him Singulair. Once more we woke to Eden's shrill cries.

When I suggested this cause-and-effect relationship to Doctor Anderson, she told me that she had never heard of such a side effect. The only people who had were a few parents on some Internet discussion boards. They described similar behaviors in their children who were taking Singulair. Want to know what doctors love? Doctors love it when you cite anonymous postings from Internet discussion boards when you question their recommendations.

Actually, Doctor Anderson was quite gracious about my concerns. She simply hadn't heard of the side effect I described since it wasn't a circulating truth. Nonetheless, I believed that it was a truth for Eden. Being Eden's mother for three years had taught me to trust his responses, however improbable. I trusted myself. Good thing. Though I don't know when the Singulair website was updated with the information, when I checked it in 2010 among the side effects listed were bad or vivid dreams, disorientation, anxiety, hallucinations, and sleepwalking.

The problem was that, like Doctor Anderson, I wanted to control Eden's asthmatic flairs. How would Singulair have helped? Singulair is different from an antihistamine, which blocks histamines. Singulair targets chemical mediators called leukotrienes, which have powerful effects on bronchial inflammation. As compared to histamines, very small amounts of leukotrienes can cause long-lasting asthmatic reactions. So Eden's second, less effective choice after Singulair was a daily dose of antihistamine. Although Doctor Anderson suggested that Eden could take an antihistamine only during peak allergy seasons—spring and fall—I wasn't thrilled with that plan. Eden had been on Zyrtec from five to eighteen months old. He also had taken two different antacids. It was then that we had taken him off all his medications on Doctor Anderson's advice. She had been concerned that medication might mask his chronic symptoms and add confusion during a confusing time.

Then again, Eden was about to start preschool. There haven't been many studies of the relationship between school-age children, medication, and learning, but a few have indicated that whether children take what is called a first-generation antihistamine, the really drowsy kind, or a second-generation antihistamine, the less drowsy kind, the effects may reduce their ability to learn. Both the mother and the schoolteacher in me struggled with the possibility of a spaced-out schoolboy.

I had already made a point of sampling all of Eden's medicines to understand how he might have felt. His potencies were too low for me to feel any effects. Instead, I learned tastes. Eden's first Zyrtec bottle was wild cherry Life Savers with a hint of nickel. His next prescription, custom-compounded, unflavored, dye-free Zyrtec, was sugary diluted library paste. Eden's first antacid, prescribed for his reflux, had underlying notes of dental tooth polish. His second antacid was tannic grape. None of it tasted good to me, but I had given it to him nonetheless in syringes, spoons, and cups.

My dilemma was compounded by other concerns. During the year preceding Eden's first asthma attack, his developmental therapists let me know that he was closing in on the fully functional three-year-old finish line. I agreed. I lived his progress, watched his confidence grow. And as I did, it was obvious that his chronic physical discomforts (itching, chronic congestion, and a smattering of random swellings) were a persistent distraction. Then, with his therapists gone, I didn't want Eden's history to repeat itself, his fearful allergic doppelgänger to resurface just as he had learned to welcome new sensations into his life. So in the year before Eden's asthma emerged, the same year we rented our off-season house, I explored alternative medical treatments. My logic? It was vague. Alternative medicine is said to be "holistic." I wasn't hoping for an alternative cure for Eden's allergies. I just wanted his body and mind to continue to communicate and play nice.

My cousins had exposed me to alternative medicine. Growing up, my ongoing fantasy was that my cousins Lisa and Debbie were my biological sisters who just happened to live in New Hampshire. (The adults had worked it out for whatever reasons.) When my cousins drove to meet us at our grandparents' apartment in Brooklyn, we fell into easy routines. We practiced headstand splits and French braided one another's hair. We hid under makeshift blanket tents hung between our grandparents' twin beds and slid Dippin' Stix into their paper pouches of tart sugar. Then we stuck our heads out into the light long enough to check whether our tongues were bleeding from the scraping from the candy. If the adults continued ignoring us, we scrounged yarn out of my grandmother's knitting basket for a finale of cat's cradle and Jacob's ladder. Oh, I loved them.

Lisa first turned to alternative medicine when the best specialists at the Lahey Clinic in Burlington, Massachusetts, couldn't solve an inner-ear problem that had all but disassembled her young adult life. Through various routes she wound up at the Omega Institute, a center for holistic health studies, where she conquered her health issues in time for motherhood. Both Lisa and Debbie continued to use alternative treatments for their families.

Ben had provided me with a short list of alternative therapies on our first visit. His list was both child-centric and esoteric since Eden, because of his unusual allergies and young age, wasn't a candidate for some typical options, such as acupuncture. I didn't think I could stand the sight of needle topography in Eden's soft flesh. Herbalists worried me too. Herbs were too close to food. Among our contenders were a technique called Namudripad's Allergy Elimination Technique (NAET), Craniosacral Therapy, osteopathy, and homeopathy.

Ben described NAET as "a sort of fusion of acupressure and kinesiology." Oh, *that*. When Drew and I researched NAET, we came across a detailed description of a patient who was cured of an egg allergy in part by having eggs placed on his stomach during treatment. Besides the fact that it sounded wacked, the only center for what we renamed the Egg on the Stomach Thing was at least an hour away.

I decided to bring Eden to a craniosacral therapist first. Craniosacral therapists use one of many osteopathic methods to apply gentle manual pressure to the skull, spine, and other areas to ease nerve passages and restore the flow of fluids throughout the brain, the spinal cord, and the surrounding membranes. The craniosacral therapist told me that Eden didn't need her therapy because he didn't have notable nerve restrictions anywhere. Done.

Next I tried a Canadian-trained osteopath named Sonia. I didn't know what an osteopath was. I found out that in the United States they are physicians who complete four years of basic medical training at osteopathic medical schools. They hold the degree doctor of osteopathic medicine (DO) as opposed to an MD degree. After medical school, like MDs, DOs obtain graduate education and training, which can last anywhere from three to eight years and allows them to practice in a specialty area such as pediatrics, family medicine, or surgery. DOs obtain state licenses and practice in licensed health-care facilities.

After reviewing the training and protocol described in the American Osteopathic Association's literature, I discovered that Sonia wasn't a U.S.-board-certified DO. She was a Canadian-trained osteopath and also a U.S.-certified physical therapist. Osteopathic practitioners educated outside the United States are known as osteopaths, not DOs, and their practices are limited to osteopathic manipulations and don't incorporate all of the techniques utilized by American DOs.

In Sonia's waiting room a flow of French-speaking mothers had lilting tones, which quieted my monkey-mind doubts about being there. After taking a careful medical history, Sonia sat Eden upright on a treatment table without his shirt. Her office was lined with shelves of glass tubes holding clear substances. They all looked the same but were labeled with different codes. She touched Eden's back, gave him a tube to hold, and then touched his back more as he held groups of glass tubes on his lap, in his hands, and sometimes against his legs. If there were too many tubes for Eden to manage, I held the tubes against his thighs.

"They just need to be touching his skin." *Mais oui.*

While Eden held the tubes, Sonia's fingers tapped over him with swift, fluttering presses as if he were a piano. Sometimes she drew on his back with a pen, creating an undecipherable chart on his pale skin that faded after a bath. When she was finished, she removed the tubes and gave them back to him one by one to hold as she touched his head. Then we sorted each tube into two piles: "Yes" and "No . . . still no."

I decided that I didn't need to understand exactly what Sonia was doing. My head was filled with other concrete details of Eden's condition, and I figured that my grasp of this treatment wasn't going to affect its efficacy. Once Sonia had waved her tapered fingers at her rows of tubes and said something like "Everything. All that we take in, that we *know*, is in those, is *there*," I surmised that the tubes held distilled versions of everyday substances, maybe even food. I guessed that she was trying to get his body to accept those substances and that maybe she was working against some resistance she felt in his skin.

"I think Sonia is kind of egg on the stomachish but without the egg," I confessed to Drew after about two months of sessions.

"I know exactly what you mean." (Clearly, we weren't getting out enough those days.)

Most important, when I asked Eden how he felt while we were walking home, he usually said "good" or "tired" or "good but tired."

Then, within about ten treatments, snap, snap, Eden's eczema retreated. It was the real deal, the thunderclap, the drumroll, and the rainbow overhead occurrence that hadn't been predicted or promised. Eden's rashes cleared within the month. *Gone.* For weeks afterward I inspected his limbs at all sorts of inappropriate and random moments, in the elevator, on the swings, and on the street. I was incredulous. For the first time in years, I could stroke him without the fear that I would tickle the itch and start his scratch cycle. I checked. I stroked. His skin had turned into butter and silk.

Eden went to Sonia for about a year. His third birthday passed. Our little weekend house, however temporary, iced our cake. And then. Then. Just as it was all getting easier, we were back home with one expired rental lease, one hospital bill, and our asthma medications. You can't die from eczema. He got worse. Asthma is worse.

After discovering Singulair's supposedly singular effect on Eden, I stopped giving it to him. His inhaled medications were for flare-ups, not daily prevention. Sonia offered to continue to treat Eden but admitted that she didn't know how much impact her treatments would have. Then there was another unwelcome surprise. Our pediatrician, Ben, moved away. He would return on occasion for special consults and left all his patients with specific referrals that were based on our needs. He also sent his patients a detailed Ben-like good-bye letter concluding with his truth: "Life has been interfering with living well." Like the rest of his patients, Drew and I were teary. He was truly unique. We found another kind and focused pediatrician, but she wasn't prone to unconventional solutions the way Ben was.

I thought. I watched and listened for the classic asthmatic signals: audible wheezes and pulling, a visible drawing of the ribs inward to take a breath. I considered two more alternative doctors. Both were doctors of osteopathic medicine. One of them was a little famous. He had published two books on the subject of allergies and nutrition, and he was Don Draper handsome, flashing a star-quality smile in his photos. His books were informative and filled with nutritional advice. I'll call him Doctor Smile.

I learned about the other DO from a friend who had taken her daughter to him years earlier. This DO's treatment had helped her daughter immediately. She told me that this doctor's son had severe multiple food allergies. She thought he had cured all of them. Part of me wished she hadn't told me that part.

I visited both doctors by myself. I had an ace-in-the-hole medical issue of my own and decided to use it as a test. My medical condition was called Raynaud's syndrome, and like Eden's allergies, it was a chronic autoimmune disorder. When I was twenty-one, a few of my fingers turned bloodless white after a summer day in the ocean. I didn't think much about it until the next winter when I studied abroad, in England, and came back to New York with frostbite damage on my toes. For years, my Raynaud's syndrome has caused my toes and fingers to turn whitish yellow and sometimes nearly blue from the slightest temperature drop. Reaching into freezers, air-conditioning, and even cool rainy days trigger extreme reactions. Simple tasks such as turning my keys and tying shoelaces were nearly impossible during Raynaud's flairs, but I never took medication because I was told that the medicines could have long-term side effects. Instead, I tried to keep my feet and hands warm and gave up winter sports. I still had Raynaud's, and so Eden didn't need to do the rounds.

Doctor Smile didn't meet with patients in person on the first visit. Policy. Waiting, I studied bottles of macadamia oil lining a display in his reception area. In his literature he referred to "miracle oil," but in light of Eden's allergies, I sat there and thought up names such as scary oil, bad oil, and very bad scary oil. After I met with Doctor Smile's nurse practitioner, she told me my blood tests confirmed Raynaud's syndrome. Yep. She recommended a vitamin therapy plus one or more treatments from specialists who worked in the same office—a group approach. I had a few concerns: I didn't see any children while I was there; after Eden's experiences with pediatric groups, I wasn't crazy about the group approach in any circumstances; and if he was too busy to meet with first-time patients, whose expertise was being utilized? After ponging between Eden's doctors, I had a better gauge on what we each needed as patient and parent.

The second osteopath, Doctor Jacobs, practiced solo, with one secretary at his front desk. The waiting room was worn but not shabby, with a few toys, and many books. I didn't wait. I've since learned that he adheres to a meticulous schedule and refuses to overbook patients. He was board-certified in osteopathic family practice, osteopathic manipulative medicine, and homeopathy. And that last one, homeopathy, is important.

Homeopathy emerged in nineteenth-century Germany, promoted by a physician and chemist named Samuel Hahnemann. As he was translating medical papers, Hahnemann read that the bitter properties of Peruvian bark accounted for its effectiveness against malaria. He proved that claim incorrect by preparing a bitter remedy from another substance that turned out to be useless against malaria. Then he tested the effects of Peruvian bark by taking small doses and eventually got the symptoms of malaria.

Hahnemann theorized that the bark was curative because it could create symptoms similar to those of malaria. By studying the records of accidental poisonings from popular medicines (mercury, arsenic, and silver nitrate), he found that an overdose of those substances corresponded to symptoms of the disease—too much of the remedy was bad, but less of it could be good. Hahnemann then coined the Latin phrase *Similia similibus curantur*—"Let likes be cured with likes."

There is evidence of the *similia* concept in conventional medicine. Immunizations protect the body through the injection of small doses of agents that cause the illness. But that's an inexact comparison to homeopathy. Unlike the one size fits all approach of immunizations, Hahnemann developed a practice from the identification of a remedy that was based on an individual's total physical and psychological characteristics. Homeopathic remedies are drawn from hundreds of substances, including herbs, flowers, minerals, elements, and even animals. Sometimes people refer to homeopathic remedies as herbs, but that definition isn't correct. Homeopathic substances are isolated and diluted to such a degree that according to conventional science, they cannot have any medicinal effect. However, according to homeopathic theory, those substances, when administered correctly, can have a powerful curative impact.*

---

*Homeopaths follow the logic that an individual's symptoms guide the remedy, which stimulates a force rather than eradicating the symptom.

Homeopathy is the most widely used form of alternative medicine in the world. According to the World Health Organization (WHO), approximately 500 million people worldwide receive homeopathic treatment. In France approximately 40 percent of the public has used homeopathic remedies, and almost half of Dutch physicians consider homeopathic remedies effective. By contrast, in the United States, at the end of the twentieth century, the American Medical Association (AMA) Code of Medical Ethics prohibited AMA members from consulting with homeopathic physicians. There was declining interest in it until the 1970s, when it experienced a resurgence and became especially popular in Europe. According to the World Health Organization, homeopathy is the second largest system of medicine in the world and is experiencing an annual growth rate of around 20 to 25 percent. My cousins had used homeopaths with great success, so there I was.

Doctor Jacobs's eyes penetrated through his thickly framed glasses as I stepped into the office. There was no hint of Ben's wide-eyed enthusiasm or Sonia's gentle accents. He was very serious during our initial interview, which I would learn later was spurred by his desire to help patients in critical need. He saved his humor for the children and those with whom he developed a rapport. Doctor Jacobs asked me many questions, and when I didn't answer to his satisfaction, he repeated the main question. "Let me put it this way. You say your fingers go from white to red. But if you don't run hot water over your fingers, then what colors do they turn?" Exactitude is a homeopath's calling card. He typed my answers into a laptop and prescribed my first homeopathic remedy.

As he pulled open a cabinet to measure the remedy into a small white envelope, he explained, "Generally, for a chronic condition I suggest a follow-up. When you begin to feel significant progress, the time between visits becomes longer and longer. It can take several years, but you should keep having improvement."

When I got home, I poured a mouthful of sweet tiny white pellets into my mouth. My feet throbbed strangely for a few nights. It was the summer, a difficult time to gauge Raynaud's syndrome, but the throbbing was interesting. Different. Later that week, when I wore sandals in a cold grocery store, my toes didn't become numb. That was different too. I decided to return.

During my second appointment, I explained Eden, giving ample room for Doctor Jacobs to prod me for elaboration. But he let me finish without interruption before answering, "My son had the same kind of allergies. Just as many. I can help your son. It took several years for mine to work his way through all his foods. Now he's in college, and sure, if he eats a few peanuts, he gets mildly itchy. So he avoids them. It's nothing serious." He paused and without a smidgen more emotion went on. "Now, if I'm successful, some people will probably tell you that Eden will have outgrown his allergies anyway in that time. People like to believe that."

Doctor Jacobs's dispassion might have made me uneasy a year earlier, but I wanted honesty. And talent. Talent in the form it might take in this medical context. Those were my priorities. His son's photograph was to the side of his large wooden desk. Who has the guts to treat his own child for anaphylactic allergies? You'd have to be either crazy or very confident. I know parents who corner doctors with this question: "What would you do if it were your child?" I didn't have to ask because the answer was framed in the face of this doctor's smiling teenager. This father believed that what he did worked. I wanted to bring Eden.

Eden's treatments were easy enough. Every appointment, Doctor Jacobs asked me questions about Eden's health and fleshed out any previous concerns, and then he determined a remedy. The only part I didn't like was that sometimes Doctor Jacobs wanted to know about things that seemed irrelevant. For example, Eden had a generally sensitive stomach. As I elaborated on a recent spell of his bothersome stomachaches, Doctor Jacobs interrupted: "What's with his lips? Are they always that dry?" Or if Eden had a stubborn bout of asthma, he might ask, "Tell me again. Is he allergic to fish?" (His question led to the search for appropriate fish oil for Eden to take medicinally.) It took a while, but eventually I saw his overriding goal. As an osteopath and homeopath, Doctor Jacobs considered Eden's sum total even as he considered a single problem. He classified illnesses as acute and chronic and addressed both.

For example, people with allergies often produce more mucus when they get a head cold. Eden was no exception, and often his lungs got so congested over a night's sleep that come morning, he would have to hack the worst of it out before he could do anything else. It was awful to witness. When Eden was that clogged up, I would take him to Doctor Jacobs for Osteopathic Manipulative Treatment (OMT). Sometimes, to alleviate the lung congestion, Doctor Jacobs would have Eden would lie on his back while he placed his hands on my son's thoracic cage (it looks like the area between the ribs) and compressed it up and down. The impression was of a lifeguard pumping a drowned person's lungs. The first time I saw it, I half expected a spout of water to come out of Eden's mouth like one of those cherubic statues in a fountain. Instead, I would notice Eden's feet: during thoratic pumping his feet would push out from his ankles in rhythm with his pumping ribs. The treatment encouraged Eden's lungs to drain. Doctor Jacobs also prescribed homeopathic remedies to complement the OMT and treat the virus. His treatments were more orchestrated than administered.

Once I saw Eden's asthma and overall stamina improve, I returned for Dayna and myself. Why? I wanted to deal with the bane of every busy parent: the horrible, terrible, very bad childhood colds and flu that keep kids out of school and parents out of work. They could disrupt the whole family when they reared their ugly virus heads just as you boarded a plane, got into a car, sat down to Christmas dinner, or left for a wedding.

Doctor Jacobs could actually make them go away by recommending the right homeopathic remedy.

So many parents are familiar with this scenario: Eden feels tired one afternoon and shortly thereafter passes out on the couch in the middle of *Hannah Montana*, a show he usually watches with unflinching intensity. I carry him to bed wondering what the morning will bring, and when he wakes with a telltale flush and runny nose, imagine me telling myself that a day of rest and fluids should do the trick. Instead, Eden's flush turns into "hot ouchy legs," and he begins to have a hacking cough. I barely leave my two-bedroom apartment for about three days. Then, on the fourth day, Dayna tells me that she's really tired and her throat feels hot.

At this point most parents feel like weeping, but they don't because they are too busy rinsing the ring of Tylenol residue out of the bottom of a plastic measuring cup or trying to figure out how they are going to work the next day. But in those situations Doctor Jacobs is able to devise a homeopathic remedy to lessen the worst symptoms and get my children's homebound bodies off the couch. No miracle quackery for me; our good doctor would also recommend rest and chicken soup—common sense. And he tests my children for secondary infections such as strep throat in order to prescribe antibiotics as needed.

Osteopaths use medicine. Selectively. Thoughtfully. In fact, Doctor Jacobs has repeatedly justified the potency, effects, and necessity of Eden's inhaled asthma medications and encourages me to administer them if other remedies aren't helping Eden enough. I have a tendency to hesitate. Eden progressed from having moderate episodic asthma every few weeks to having mild bouts every few months. He hasn't ever had to take the strong stuff—the liquid steroid prednisone.

Eden is eight, and as I write this, he is still allergic to milk, soy, some beans, sesame seeds, salmon, and of course nuts and peanuts. He seems to have outgrown some of his shellfish and fish allergies, but we have only tried one variety of each. And he can eat hard-boiled eggs but can't comfortably tolerate stovetop-cooked eggs or foods with added egg whites. Eden is allergic to plant pollen and mold, and he had a reaction to a sulfa-based antibiotic two years ago.

Every year, Drew and I take Eden back to his allergist, Doctor Anderson, and every year she tests his blood to see if he is showing clinical signs of outgrowing his allergies. I rely on Doctor Anderson for her vast knowledge of current research and medical advances. She treats hundreds of children like Eden every year, and I value her perspective. But I rely on Doctor Jacobs's as well to get us through our days. He knows our stories. He knows Eden always craves salt; Dayna will play dumb at his jokes, twisting her face into pleased mock confusion; and I rough myself up for my mistakes when in fact I'm getting smarter about my children's allergies and viruses, sometimes successfully giving them remedies at home. My Raynaud's syndrome got better too. The first winter under Doctor Jacobs's treatment I didn't need to sleep in thick socks as I had for years. My feet and fingers have had fewer episodes of numbing every season. Balancing our positive experience is the simple fact that our insurance covers only a percentage of the cost of our visits to Doctor Jacobs after we reach our deductible limits, because he isn't within our insurance network. Regular visits to an osteopath may not be a financial option for every parent, and this may create a self-fulfilling lack of evidence for the benefits.

Eventually, Doctor Jacobs shared his stories. "When my son was young, my wife packed up a travel cooler for everywhere. . . . Mistakes happen. . . . She once poured the wrong milk on his cereal. . . . My son had a nebulizer out of its box for years. . . . We put the stroller in the car and went to Jones Beach so he could have a day of fresh air. . . . He vomited it right up. . . . Sometimes a glass of ice water will give them more relief than anything else. . . . There will be bad days. . . ." Whether Eden is cured of his allergies or outgrows them or we can discern the difference, Doctor

Jacobs's treatment has enabled us to weather the storm of everyday living. For now that is miraculous enough.

We all have to learn to live within the confines of our bodies, and although parents can help their children find freedom within those confines, I often have to remind myself of my limits. Instead, we mothers can fall under our own spells and begin to believe we are Prospero, using our magic to protect our children and control their world. We want to believe that we wave our arms above our children's heads and raise them above fate, biology, beliefs, and expectations.

Despite all our very best parenting efforts—vitamins, rest, sports, Ritalin, homeopathy, yoga, Claritin—there are mornings many of us parents will lean over our coffee cups and listen to the distant sounds of our children waking and wonder if today will be the day their head cold or indigestion or anxiety or adenoids or teething pains or leg cramps or some other weakness will get the best of them. I'm no wizard, so I tell myself to just keep teaching Eden to cope with his allergies as I try to improve them.

Despite the very best efforts of my doctors, sometimes Eden goes to school with bothersome allergies. What does it feel like to get dressed and walk to school after sucking down two metered puffs of a bronchodilator? Well, it is much better than going to school without having done so. I tried Eden's inhaler, of course, one day after dropping him off at school. It tasted like damp chemicals. It made my heart thump at a faster rhythm than my breath, my head felt overfull of air, and I was at once energized and tired. Although it didn't diminish my appetite for breakfast, Eden's hunger is often suppressed for several hours. Eden reports the dichotomy of sensations as "buzzy and sleepy."

According to the Asthma and Allergy Foundation of America, asthma is the leading cause of school absences caused by a chronic illness. It accounts for an annual loss of more than fourteen million school days per year (approximately eight days for each student with asthma) and more hospitalizations than any other childhood disease. It has been estimated that children with asthma spend nearly eight million days per year restricted to bed, days their parents surely hadn't counted on.[22]

Like other parents, I have shaped a circle of school support—teachers, nurses, us—to help Eden face the challenges of a day spent feeling not good but not too terrible. I arm him with a plan: (1) don't hesitate to tell a teacher if you think you need to see the nurse; (2) don't panic or worry about what you are about to miss; and (3) tell the nurse whether you need medicine or just rest or water. To an adult this is an obvious sequence, not much of a big plan, but to Eden it's a formula for inner resolve, the same kind of inner resolve I saw in my student Alex.

We parents can't make magic. We can't transform our children. But we can heal with our touches, our words, and our love. We can show them how to take their medicine. When we do this, our children can save themselves.

Chapter 7

OPPOSITE DAY

In my fourth-grade class, we embraced the concept of opposite day. At least once a month we greeted each other in the schoolyard with a cheery "Good-bye, I detest you!" and then burst out with the always hilarious "Just kidding. It's opposite day!" All day long it was more of the same: "I'm so lucky to have these delicious celery sticks." "Don't you just love spelling quizzes?" Since we could speak the worst about classmates under the guise of humorous contradiction, opposite day had a cruel edge. These days, Eden's food allergies sometimes make me feel like I'm back in opposite day.

Parties are a great example of the opposite effect since they can invoke conflicted, anxious feelings for people dealing with food allergies. We learned this lesson when Eden turned two. For days Eden heard Dayna report on the upcoming celebration with its modest guest list of grandparents, cousins, and a few close friends. Dayna repeated "coming to your birthday" to Eden, her eyes opening just a fraction wider so that he would understand there was magic in her words.

I spent weeks planning the menu, leafing through new and untested recipes. I was determined not to serve even one crumb that Eden couldn't eat at his party, and so the birthday menu would be a cunning mélange of safe foods. In the days leading up to the birthday brunch, I bought several new cookbooks with titles like *Cooking without Dairy and Loving It!* and *Who Needs Nuts?* I used one of them to concoct dairy-free, egg-free, soy-free pear blondies. They baked upward in the heat of the oven and then flattened into pale defeat on the Formica counter. Undaunted, I prepared a vanilla cake that didn't deflate but shared the blondies' pallor. As I stared down, both the blondies and the cake silently pleaded like little paupers: "Please, Mum, please. Gimme chocolate then." Surely some chocolate topping would have enhanced their colorless appearance. But no, Doctor Anderson hadn't yet given me the allergy permission slip to consider that transformative ingredient. Although it doesn't rank in the "top eight" allergens—peanuts, tree nuts, dairy, soy, egg, wheat, fish, and shellfish—at the time she considered chocolate risky for Eden. He was, after all, allergic to seven out of those eight heavy hitters in addition to a few other foods.

How to help those poor cakes? I melted together a sugar and water glaze because I couldn't find a dairy- *and* soy-free shortening that would have substituted for a buttercream type of frosting. I colored the glaze with a few teaspoons of double-brewed Twinings English Breakfast tea because God knows, I wouldn't have dared to mess around with food coloring. Still, while spreading the taupe icing on the crumbly cakes, I worried about a woman I knew in college who used to get nose-pinching migraines from even the slightest amount of coffee or chocolate. Did she get headaches from tea too? I couldn't recall.

The final home-baked offering was a batch of rye breadsticks. There was a picture of the finished product in my cookbook, but I must have rolled the dough into stubbier formations. Once baked, they looked less like sticks than like half-smoked cigars or, as Drew commented, not unkindly, after glancing at the bread tray, "Ah, big turds!"

"Yep. Exactly," I answered back, not sarcastically. "But they taste all right."

The morning of the party I was up at 6 a.m. broiling a large package of Jones pork sausage links. I'd previously confirmed this with the forthcoming, nay, the jovial Jones Dairy Farm customer service representative, who assured me that the ready-to-cook package contained only meat and benign spices: "That's right, miss. Just don't purchase the oven-browned variety."

Got it! No oven-browned. As I brooded over the stove, turning the links attentively with a kitchen tong, suddenly they too looked like turds. Smaller ones. "Shit!" I muttered beneath my breath.

As planned, I sent Drew out of the apartment to pick up a Box O'Joe from the Dunkin' Donuts on First Avenue. "This!" he proclaimed upon returning, his hand gripping the white handle of the coffee carton, "is what we should be getting every morning. Forget the party!"

"You're cra-azy!" I bantered back, as if we exchanged witticisms all the time instead of monosyllabic exchanges before a child, the telephone, or the urge to fall sleep interrupted us. Like most couples, we had our warm-up routines, our ways of putting on our collective game face.

Time was short. Suddenly it was less than an hour before our guests were due to arrive, and I hadn't showered. I started the DVD of *Maisy's ABC*, and both children hustled over to the couch at the opening bars of the theme song. I rushed into the bathroom as Drew rushed out, a towel wrapped around his waist. "Done?"

"Yes!"

As the warm water pulsed against the back of my neck, I imagined the piles of food that would surely remain on everyone's paper party plate, poorly hidden under crumpled napkins: shriveled sausage links hiding under the crumbs of blondies picked apart and uneaten. Fretting, I peeked out minutes later, towel around my head. Dayna and Eden were staring ahead, motionless. There was a purple cup in Eden's hand. But I had poured his rice milk into his blue cup that morning. Definitely. The blue one.

As I pushed open the bedroom door, my words ran swift and hot. "Where did you get Eden's cup from?"

"From the counter."

At Drew's answer my knee joints buckled backward. The counter. That was where I had put Dayna's cup. The counter. Her cup was purple, and it was filled with soy milk. The word *soy* filled my brain and pressed the outer edges of my skull. S-O-Y. Then a sliver of space opened between the *o* and the *y*, and I squeezed a direction through that space. *Get it. Get—the—cup—now.* I walked to the couch, bent in supplication, held out Eden's little blue cup, and emoted in my most child-lacquered tone, "Eden . . . let's trade cups. Okay?"

"Nooo!" Eden howled abruptly. "Nooo, nooo!" He clutched the purple cup with two hands. All morning the birthday word had been floating through the air like a paper airplane just within his reach. After all, we had woken him up by saying, "It's your day, Eden!" Thus empowered, Eden rejected my cup offering with an emphatic "mine!" He pulled Dayna's purple cup back from my grasp, causing three to five small droplets to fly onto the couch, his right leg, and his right hand.

I grabbed the cup away. But as I did, Eden rubbed his eyes in an aggravated cry, and Drew and I watched as the translucent skin around his right eye puffed like a toasted marshmallow. Within seconds, red oval hives sprouted over his left cheek. It was like one of those eight-millimeter school films in which the life cycle of a plant is fast-forwarded from days into seconds.

We reacted immediately, a crisis couple, and forced a syringe of Benadryl into Eden's closed lips. As he twisted his head, we pulled up his clothes for a hive body check and ran for a cup of water (flush it!). It was enough. As quickly as it came, it went. The puffing receded, and the hives melted slowly away. By the time our guests arrived, they couldn't have seen more than a slight swelling around Eden's left eye, and only if they looked closely. Once again, we got lucky.

We didn't talk about what had just happened—Eden's hair-raising, table-turning brush with soy milk droplets—even when guests remarked on his meditative (read: medicated) behavior. Why would we? Reeling from fear and finding our balance in the middle of aftershocks, we could not bear to hear: "Well, thank God, and he looks great now!" or "Wow, really? And you'd never know it. Probably bothers you more than him at this point." Those well-intended words would have tipped us right into an abyss of emotions.

Living with Eden's allergies, Drew and I have learned that we often feel worse when people offer us encouragement. All we really want to hear is, "That must have been very scary for all you." That's it. Why? Because our fear is our most reliable truth. Parents of kids with food allergies get scared all the time. And we get especially scared of parties, holidays, vacations—in fact, all occasions that break our carefully constructed routines. Occasions that for most families implied fun and freedom opened our world to mistakes and misjudgments.

As Drew and I grapple with our adult emotions, we are humbled by Eden's challenges. Tactical miscalculations such as getting distracted by our party planning, forgetting the ice pack before a long car trip, and arriving so late to the movie theater that the only remaining seats are covered in buttery popcorn—these parental mishaps shrink compared with Eden's responsibilities. At most festivities, he is the child who must not. Reliably, he can't eat whatever's on those other twenty Batman plates neatly set out on the matching tablecloth. Eden knows better than to tug my sleeve for a handful of those ruffled potato chips or that hunk of cheddar on a side table.

We walk the line. Like other food allergy families, we have devised allergy- and travel-friendly party substitutes. Our pizza is simple: olive oil, ketchup and any hard and toasty Eden-safe bread that can absorb those condiments and remain intact. Baguettes and pita work best. We have, of course, a short list of homemade sweets to substitute for birthday cakes. Sometimes I feel bad that I'm not working myself into a sweat slicing nitrate-free pepperoni and slivers of mushrooms (so noble), but for now Eden prefers the tastes of simple foods.

The best substitutes can go only so far.

Q: How do you substitute for the choices offered during, say, a birthday party in a candy store complete with a chocolate fountain and unlimited, unlabeled confections?

A: You don't, certainly not with homemade chocolate cake. Oh, and then at Eden's first day camp there were more than a few make-your-own-sundae occasions when I prepacked sorbet surrounded by ice packs in a cooler with sandwich bags of sprinkles, minimarshmallows, and allergen-free chocolate chips. It was "uh, a little too sweet, I think," Eden said tactfully.

Although most party hopping might sound doable with a plan and a good attitude, there were parties at which I stood in the corner muttering darkly at the sight of those damn piñatas—those grinning cartoon characters that swung drunkenly, Tootsie Rolls already leaking out of their exaggerated facades. Eden would share in his peers' barbaric pleasures—the storming of the cascading candy. But after the minute-long frenzy ended, reality hit when he turned to me so flushed. Small. "What can *I* have?" At which point my heart would roll over for the seventh time that hour.

Then there are the days when I expect the worst of an occasion in which the potential for a mistake looms large, and I'm dead wrong. When Eden was in first grade, his teacher taught a social studies unit on China. The unit finished with a class trip to Chinatown to eat lunch in a Chinese restaurant. Since Eden was allergic to peanuts, soy, and sesame as well as about four other foods, the considerate preset menu that his teacher sent to the parents was immaterial to us.

Eden's teachers had been careful handling his food allergies, and so I trusted them as much as I trusted anyone, an equation that ebbs and flows with the proximity of Eden's most recent allergic "accident." After much thought, talk, and e-mailing, his teachers and I decided that Eden had two obvious options: stay back at school as a "special teacher's helper" or go with his class, toting a "safe food." Eden chose the latter. But of course he wanted his safe food to resemble the other kids' food. "Can you not pack me a sandwich, okay? Can it be like restaurant food, just mine?" Understandable. We talked further and decided that he would bring my home-cooked Chinese broccoli and eat the restaurant rice, plus he would sit next to his classroom teacher. Everything was set until I realized I had made a previous commitment to accompany my mother to a doctor's appointment and so couldn't be a class parent trip helper.

But wait. That day, that trip, was normal. Nothing happened concerning Eden's allergies. *Nothing.* Yet in preparation for a two-hour trip, I spent two hours e-mailing his teachers, discussing "the plan" with Eden, and preparing and packing his food in thermal containers. The day of the trip my brain was swishing around in its bubble of worries. The possibilities ranged from Eden's hurt feelings from being the odd man out with his broccoli to images of sesame oil and soy sauce sliding onto his fingers and then into his itchy eyes. But again, the only palpable difference that day was my fear of what could happen, a momentary fear in Eden's growing life.

Along with Eden's close calls, we are from time to time confronted with a particular kind of emotional vulnerability, a vulnerability unique to a young child whose food restrictions affect his identity. A few months after Eden's Chinatown excursion, one of his school plays had a very different outcome. Yet the event began so lightheartedly.

Like his classmates, Eden had rehearsed for weeks, practicing his lines, singing along to the DVD, and fretting over every detail of his costume. His first-grade rendition of the Robert Lopshire picture book *Put Me in the Zoo* promised a wholesome bite of childhood for all us parents to savor for years to come. The play was based on the story of a leopard who wants to live in a zoo, but the zoo doesn't want him. He goes about convincing a little boy and a girl that with "all the things he can do" the zoo is where he belongs. Eventually, the children convince the leopard that he will be a perfect fit in a circus. It works out nicely.

Eden's ego was pumped the morning of the performance when he reminded me, "Mommy, remember there's a play party in a room right after." Whoops. Since I had stopped attending Dayna's class parties, I had not remembered Eden's class specifically. But my entire morning schedule was clear.

"Of course I remembered. What substitutes do you want me to bring?"

Before I could reel off the options, Eden answered, "Nah. I'll be okay. Usually at the parent stuff they just have muffins and bagels." His nonchalance wasn't surprising. By age seven, he could pretty well predict when an occasion might be stocked with tantalizing fare as opposed to his go-to alternatives such as cut fruit or an unseeded, unadorned, unbuttered bagel. Besides, his teacher kept a stash of Oreos for the plethora of half and whole birthday parties they celebrated there. I figured that even if he called the wrong shot, we had sufficient backup.

The play? Of course it was a shiny performance. Still tingling with the warm excitement of Eden's bright future in the performing arts, I tromped up five flights holding his hand and opened the classroom door to IT. IT was a cake. But no, it was more than just a cake, it was a *cake sculpture*, a high-ranking contender in a Food Network pastry competition, a mountain of chiseled frosting (literally a mountain) covered in lions and tigers and bears. Oh, my! There were edible palm trees and jungle vegetation at the base, and each tier was toppling with spun sugar and buttercream. And like a demonically sweet centrifuge, the cake had rings of children and parents remarking on and fawning over it.

What was such a cake doing there without my knowledge? Clearly, I had miscalculated by failing to touch base with the class mother who had ordered the cake. I had a self-flagellating, stomach-churning moment followed by the realization that Eden probably felt worse than I did. Eden had a remarkable poker face, so I had to guess first. Bending, smiling, casual, I asked him if he wanted to check out the rest of the refreshments. He nodded, so we filled his plate with a bagel and two slices of cantaloupe.

Back at our table (conveniently located next to the cake), I sat down next to Eden, knees up to my chin, and listened quietly while he whispered (as if you could hear anything in the ongoing cake-cutting, ogling, plate-thrusting mayhem) that he just wondered "what it tasted like, you know?" He stared into me, his gray-green eyes pools of sadness. Maybe I was wrong. Maybe I wasn't.

My answer came out like this: "Know what? Bet it's kind of bad . . . actually." To which I got an accomplice's smirk.

Encouraged, I went on: "In fact, I bet it's the kind of cake that has grainy, yucky icing, you know, the kind where there are all those weird bumps on your tongue." (Eden had no idea what I was referring to, but it hardly mattered.) "And the batter part is probably all dried out just so the cake can stay up so high." To which I got a giggle. And that was when I began going hog-wild. Snout flying in the air, I gambled: "I bet that cake would be so, so bad that it would make us burp so loud and we would want to throw it down the toilet and flush it!"

Dear God, I was unstoppable. I had just used toilet talk (complete with the word *toilet*) to lift my seven-year-old's spirit. But Eden's real smile had returned. He was chuckling. I went on: I used the G word (*gross*); I clowned out "ewwws"; and I bent to iCarly-level witticism: "Helloo, peep-ul! It's just a *cake*!" I whispered into his ear. I said awful things about that cake. I was a terrible, horrible, no-good role model of civility. Anyone listening might have been tempted to put me in the zoo or even the circus, but as I sat in the bull's-eye of that cake, my sorrow and Eden's burden, taking aim with those very bad words was all I could do. I was tired of opposite day.

Does Eden get tired of having food allergies? Yes. Yes, he does. If you ask, he might say, "Yeah. Used to it." But time and again his disappointment and his food envy are tangible, just as clear as my memories of his allergic reactions. His food envy is often unpredictable, much like our frustrations. "They just smell so *good*," he remarks about the cafeteria French fries one Tuesday out of twenty. "Everyone had so *many* things on their plate," he comments after Thanksgiving dinner. Thankfully, like many parents who have children with medical differences, I've spent more time being amazed by Eden's practiced stride than blotting tears and offering fresh solutions and hugs in the aftermath of parties and holidays.

Opposite day was one reason I found a local support group. Kathy Franklin was a coleader of a group named PAAC (Parents of Allergic and Asthmatic Children). Her son's throat closed seventeen years earlier after he *touched* an egg noodle. Back then, who would have believed it? Many didn't. Kathy was among the first parents and patients the media identified to illustrate the rise in the prevalence of food allergies. As long ago as 2001, the *New York Times* ran a feature called "The Allergy Prison," which was the first of many articles about food allergies. In it, several members of my support group described their experiences.

I called Kathy a few months after I began seeing Doctor Reiss. I was encouraged by my experience of talk therapy, hashing out solutions to specific problems. Kathy was reassuring during our first phone call. As I introduced myself, Eden, his allergies, and our situation, she must have heard something in my voice to make her say, "It's not your fault, you know. You do know that, right?" I did. I did. I understood it. Still, many days, if even for a minute, my thoughts scanned the years of bottles, meals, and decisions, looking for some mistake there.

Kathy must have understood the futility of such guilt. She kept me in the present. She told me her son was about to start college. He had outgrown his egg allergy when he was fourteen, but he had a sesame and nut allergy that he hadn't outgrown. In a dry, deep voice Kathy related anecdotes of her life with her son. She knew exactly what I needed to hear. Her son went to coffee shops with high school friends and ate hamburgers on English muffins instead of buns. He cooked a lot now—he had taken an understandable interest in making his own food.

More information: "Once in a while he screwed up. You have to let them live. He had to go the emergency room a few times in high school." We moved on to the logistics of holidays and special events. Kathy summed up what I was already beginning to suspect: "You're probably going to want to pass on some occasions. We did. But it made our family really close." She added, "Oh. But don't miss our next meeting because it's our last of the season since we don't meet over the summer."

That meeting was in a member's home on the Upper West Side, though we usually meet in the medical offices of our attending allergist. I walked into a long living room filled with chairs set in an oval. To the side was a table with trays of peanut-, tree nut–, seed-, and dairy-free minimuffins and a fruit salad studded with red grapes. A round of introductions followed.

"You guys know me. I'm Stacy, and my six-year-old daughter, Lea, has peanut, tree nut, egg, soy, and shellfish. We've been to the emergency room twice. The first time she was just a baby."

"She's milk, corn, peanuts, peas. Now we think seeds too . . ."

"Hi. We were diagnosed three months ago. I'm Laura, and my son is Josh. He's wheat, nuts, and milk . . ."

Every parent had a list of foods and a list of unforgettable reactions. A few of the children who were discussed seemed to enjoy easy health despite their food allergies. Others sounded like Eden. Not sick but uncomfortable, kids with irritating bodies that got in their way. One child had a chronic eye condition. Skin sensitivities abounded. Asthma cavorted through that room.

As I listened, I found moorings, places I might weigh anchor with Eden. The group discussed school issues, camps, and camp nurses. They analyzed the new food labeling laws. "What's with *may* contain? Should I assume it *does?*"

A woman wearing a pink angora sweater offered a travel tip: "I use those tiny shampoo bottles for meds instead of the sample-size ones. Those sample bottles get that crust around the neck. Once I couldn't get his Benadryl open when I needed it." She blinked rapidly, remembering.

Another mother had just made a short video of herself explaining her son's condition. The previous year, after his first year of middle school, she discovered that it was too time-consuming for all his teachers to speak to her individually about his allergies. "He had so many different classes! And they don't give you much time."

After introductions, conversation flowed. We went around the room, bringing up concerns. Our attending doctor fielded the medical questions. Kathy fielded the general questions, and others volunteered personal tips: I tried to tell the program director. I don't even try. We're going to the hospital next month. The teacher said. I said. I say he can't be near it. He just can't. Always have it with you. He put his medicine in his suitcase. That didn't work for us. She thought she could handle it. Came on so suddenly.

I braced myself for Eden's future while submerged in my present reality. It was all there in that room.

Toward the end of the meeting, we learned the results of some food trials with heated milk. Then Kathy announced, "We're trying to get Doctor Sampson to come to a meeting soon. I'm thinking maybe we can send questions ahead." She didn't bother to explain who he was. He was a leading food allergy research doctor at Mount Sinai, and we all knew that. Doctor Sampson had been working toward finding a remedy for the worst offender—the peanut allergy—for years. Between 1997 and 2002 the number of children with fatal peanut allergies doubled. Between 1997 and 2008 the number of fatal peanut and tree nut allergies in children tripled, according to one survey. In the United States and Europe, peanuts and tree nuts are the most commonly reported foods to cause life-threatening reactions. In 2009, 1.5 percent of the U.S. population (about 4.5 million people) were reported to be allergic to peanuts.

As group members suggested meeting spaces large enough to host Doctor Sampson and the expected crowd, Kathy joked, "We'll need a concert hall. He's like a rock star to us."

After I left the meeting, those words pulled me back in time to the first apartment Drew and I shared. It was his apartment, but I moved in in time to finish off the rental lease. A vacuous duplex in a remodeled East Village prewar, it was so not us. Drew was trapped in his first job, and I was substitute teaching. He wore suits, and my formal wardrobe consisted of some threadbare J.Crew separates. We were pretty sure this wasn't who we were meant to be. Industrial and irregularly shaped, the apartment reflected our confusion. It had a gigantic structural pillar smack in the middle of the living room. And we had a surplus of artistic-looking neighbors who wore stiff high suede boots and leather jackets and owned dogs in extra large. I guessed they hung funky tapestries and nude photos on that pillar while our postcollege IKEA couches unartistically jutted around it to accommodate television viewing. But the coolest neighbor by far was David Lee Roth. He lived only a few floors above us, and we loved that. We even got to share the elevator with him a few times, sinking down to the lobby faux-casually, soaking in his fame. As I walked to the subway that night of my first meeting, I thought about how motherhood had reinvented my idols. There was a time when rock stars were my rock stars.

I probably attended two or three more support meetings by myself over the next school year. Drew had just started his own company; the four of us had shared endless winter flu and a spring stomach virus. By May, I was desperate for Drew to see what the support group was like, so we cleared the evening for the year-end meeting. We both needed a boost. Recent misunderstandings with family and friends over Eden's allergies were eating away at us. As we passed a box of Entenmann's cookies from lap to lap, a mother on my right told a story. She was bitterly disappointed with her extended family. While cooperatively planning a party for her parents' twenty-fifth anniversary, she had been consulted on nearly everything—except for the presence of "literally a bowl of mixed nuts sitting on every side table. Indoors and out!" She had attended with her tree-nut-allergic son and husband.

We, being her support group, murmured, "Just didn't think!" and "So many other foods!" We knew why she felt misunderstood. The problem wasn't that she couldn't keep her son away from the colonies of nut bowls. The problem was that it's hard to spend a celebratory evening anxiously hanging near a toddler in case he decides to lick the salt off the Planters Honey Roasted Mixed Nuts. And why would anyone, your family members especially, want to make your life harder so that they could serve bowls of nuts?

Of course I had to overthink it and wonder why her family would even want nuts in the face of champagne and other typical fancy party treats. Even a roasted macadamia (how good are macadamias?) wasn't as distinctive as a phyllo pastry puff filled with spinach and goat cheese or maybe some salty pancetta wrapped around a chunk of sweet honeydew. Silently, I answered myself with "what if?" instead of "why?" A guest may possibly drop a cashew at the allergic boy's feet. He steps on it and grinds the meat into his rubber sole. Cashews are fairly soft nuts, so once home, as he tiredly pulls off his shoes, some of the nut particles get on his hands and under his nails, which he has a habit of biting. What then? While the others talked pain and anger, I explored every nuance of the mother's story, every pitfall. Then their voices receded.

I pulled away from the group behind my wall of silent, vague dread. I had had this feeling before, but it was different that evening. A part of me stayed there with Drew and the others, grounded and waiting while I let myself go, really go. I went to where it was the worst. I went to the edge of that mother's cliff where her son was gasping, inflating, reaching his arms out to her. And her son was Eden, and we were running, running so hard and fast to get medicine, to get help, to escape a horror that could explode and then saturate my entire world until nothing would ever look the same again.

Except for Drew. Drew was sitting there by my side, and he looked exactly the same as he always had, as I believed he always would. We had that. He squeezed my arm. The story frightened him too. Every time we consider what can happen to Eden, really consider it, we shake off our fears and move on. I attend my support group so I can return to my family stronger, ready again. After five years, I'm able to lend some insight to new members. I'm not as sage as Kathy or the other veterans, but the new parents' challenges are still fresh. I can recognize their deer-in-the-headlights worries and doubts as my own.

When a child is diagnosed with life-threatening food allergies, new parents will come to our group with at least one upsetting story from before that diagnosis. I believe that those parents will always have their memories of a chronically sick baby or a toddler swollen with an allergic reaction, but those images will be pushed aside eventually. Often new parents can't believe (especially if the allergic child is their first) that one day their child will, for example, learn to snap his fingers. When Eden taught himself to snap, for a brief three weeks of second grade, he snapped all the time. When he spoke, his jazzy snapping marked every word. It was like conversing with a mini Frank Sinatra. Or their allergic children will learn to do something else—they will juggle two tennis balls, or rap their words into song, or memorize the choreography of their favorite pop star dancing in a YouTube video. Then those parents will let go of their fears a little bit more, and it will become that much easier for them to do what they have to do. We need to be afraid, but not too much.

Years after I brought Eden to the emergency room for the first time and the attending doctor warned, "Don't get crazy," I listened and then reassured another tearful mother as she described her recent encounter with an emergency medical technician (EMT). He had made her feel foolish and weak by chiding her for failing to use her EpiPen on her son. She was too scared to put that needle into his flesh, so she called the paramedics. She froze, feeling she might do more harm than good. (Our attending allergist told her she was incorrect.) The group spent the remainder of that evening injecting oranges with expired EpiPens, practicing with her and building her confidence, because we were there to help one another help our children in the most literal and the most abstract sense of that word.

A child with serious food allergies can unwittingly make his or her parents feel like there is an electric fence encircling their home. Leave the perimeter and you might get shocked, jolted backward. When I break from routines, there is always a risk particular to Eden. Whether I hire a new babysitter, purchase a new brand of tortillas, or plan a family day trip by ferry, all reasonable actions, I chance the unforeseeable.

When it was still age-appropriate, I solved the question of Eden's safety on playdates simply by inviting his friends to our home. If the playdate had to be in someone else's home because of logistics or the lure of that child's particular game or toy, I stayed there, bringing books to occupy myself. Then, when Eden started second grade, he began to feel a little stifled by my approach. "Mom, no offense, but I want to go to Nick's house on, like, a *drop-off*." So we began taking steps toward independence. I've started to leave Eden with his bag of medicine, snacks, and instructions to the parent. I'm selective depending on the distance, the time span, and the supervision. For example, when one mother told me her husband is diabetic and so she was very comfortable administering all of Eden's medicines, Eden had carte blanche to play there anytime.

Another parent worried me because she insisted, "I know all about allergic food because my nephew is allergic to peanuts," and so I repeated to her that Eden could eat only from his snack bag. No exceptions. And Eden wants to stay safe. Thus far, he has been self-regulating in school situations and otherwise. When he has even the slightest doubt about a food, he passes. Often Eden asks us to taste a food or beverage for him as an extra precaution. Eden understands his comfort zone: at eight years old, he hasn't attended a birthday party without either Drew or me staying on because he's told us he doesn't feel ready.

Travel is another gamble. For the food-allergic, even tame Berenstain Bears–style vacations are fertile ground for unpredictable moments and poor decisions hastened by the words "let's just stop here for lunch; I'm sure we'll find something safe." In a blink, there I am, stupidly allowing my still hungry but still allergic child to pick at the unlabeled, unidentifiable pita out of the bread basket since the chef charred his grilled hamburger into an inedible hockey puck and my other child isn't done with her grilled cheese. (For some reason I have found that the words *food allergy* often inspire cooks to overcook, as if they can burn off any of the offending foods.) That is why, when Eden was first diagnosed, I assumed that the complete Weissman family unit would not be leaving our tristate area for years to come.

And indeed, at the beginning, the four of us rarely strayed. Sure, I brought Dayna to visit with her second cousins in New Hampshire. We left Drew and Eden to fend for themselves in the wilds of Manhattan with a stack of DVDs higher than my waist and preplanned, preshopped, nearly prechopped menu plans. Sure, we rented two nearby houses so that our children would understand that yards weren't fictitious geography. And of course Drew traveled, mostly to the West Coast, for work. But after almost three years of allergic near-lockdown and long New York winters, I began to feel like a scaredy-cat. Drew and I craved the freedom and fun of sunshine in February and the pleasure of our children's pleasure.

But where to go? If Eden was going to expect a reasonable caloric intake while on vacation, I needed a fully operational kitchen, not a kitchenette. He was a growing and hungry toddler. As it was, I worried about running out of safe food and grappled with Eden's frustration on simple outings to the local playground. But I didn't particularly want to rent another house to spend a week cooking, cleaning, and devising kid-friendly amusements to re-create our everyday lives with better weather. I wanted my family to do something special together.

One evening at a support group meeting, someone mentioned Disney World. I began to grasp that part of the "spectacular memories" (and spectacular expense) of a Disney vacation was Disney's die-hard commitment to accommodate all kinds of children, including the highly allergic. Confession: I had never been to Disney World in Orlando, Florida. One of my grandmothers used to live in Los Angeles, so once when I was very young, we went to Disneyland for a day. All I remember is the lyrics from "It's a Small World": "It's a world of laughter and a world of tears" (so true). And I remember the horrifying moment when my balloon escaped from my mother's hand in the parking lot and she demanded that my brother "share" amid our exhausted tears. So when I began making inquiries, I was a Disney virgin with no concept of the multitude of Disney vacation options.

There were suites and villas at Disney World with more square footage than my apartment. The words *child*, *food*, and *allergy* seemed to cast a magical spell on Disney staffers. There were enchanting restaurants where the chefs were ready and able to ensure a triple-washed frying pan into which they would place lightly julienned vegetables, sauté them in olive oil, and bring them out to your food-allergic child to chitchat about the carrots. There were trip planners who happily explained the food and beverage options available at all locales and scheduled points of our Disney days.

Still, there were some small hurdles: we wanted to spend our days at the theme parks where there were no magical restaurants, just fast-food offerings replete with cross-contaminated fryer oil cooking. Hotel breakfasts were problematic and limited. Imagining those miles of Disney paths as a serious toddler calorie burn, I wanted a stove and refrigerator to prepare Eden's breakfast and takeout lunch and snacks. Some of my preparations: I booked Disney rooms with a full kitchen. I sent ahead a large box filled with dry goods such as cereal, crackers and special-order granola bars, and a loaf of bread, which turned fuzzy green in transit. Before leaving New York, I located the nearest supermarket and called about Eden's brand of rice milk because Drew was dead certain that the hermetically sealed rice milk cartons would burst in my dry goods box. Somehow we persuaded both children to spend their first morning grocery shopping. "We'll push you so fast in the cart, it'll be just like a roller coaster!"

I spoke to the managers of two restaurants ten weeks in advance of our dinner reservations. I found out that desserts were going to be a problem, so I included the ingredients for my chocolate cake in my send-ahead box. (I also threw in a few packets of instant yeast, which proved invaluable when I was confronted with the moldy mess in my bread wrapper.)

Were my efforts worthwhile? Entirely. Dayna and Eden wore a commercial and clichéd look of wonder on their faces from the moment we arrived. Their eyes got wider by the day. We shuttled between theme parks, going on every age-, weight-, and height-appropriate ride. We decided that Goofy wasn't scary but also wasn't actually goofy. Dayna decided she wasn't the "princess type." Yes, those quotation marks were gestured with appropriate finger bending and emphasis. After cruising the parks, we cooled down in the pool near our rooms. Drew and I head banged to snatches of theme park songs just to make the kids laugh. I baked bread rolls and chocolate cake in my Disney oven and toted pieces to dinner so that Dayna could order a restaurant dessert with her family. It felt like a real vacation.

When we were walking back to our rooms on the second-to-last day, Dayna spotted a small toad on the white-hot cement path. "Look! It's a frog. A toad!"

Eden chimed in: "Toad frog!"

The next day, when the children thought they saw the same toad in exactly the same spot, they began jumping and shouting, "He's back! The toad frog!"

It was the kind of scorching yet humid day that an amphibian might glory in, but Drew and I milked it. "He was waiting for you. It's him! "

Years later, whenever I ask Eden what he remembers about Disney World, he answers, "Toad Frog! Remember Toad Frog?!"

"Is that it?" I ask again. And then I tick down the list of more significant attractions. "Remember when they opened the gates at Animal Kingdom? How wet we got on the Pirates of the Caribbean?"

"Nope" . . . "No" . . . "I just remember Toad Frog."

That's how it is. Parents sweat the details of our children's pleasures. Then the children choose their memories. And sometimes, as they recall, your paradise was their Toad Frog.

Chapter 8

NEW NORMAL

I WANTED TO GO POSTAL ON SPONGEBOB for his machine gun laugh and wide pin-legged stride. Obviously, I had been cooped up in that hospital room for one episode too many. But there we were, Eden and I, our presence voluntary. No crisis for a change: we were at the tail end of a "shrimp challenge." No puns needed since the possibility that my food-allergic five-year-old might have outgrown, of all his allergies, his shrimp allergy seemed screwy enough without the timely aquatic themes of Eden's beloved television show.

For children with life-threatening allergies, food challenges are often the safest way to test whether they've outgrown a particular allergy. Food challenges are designed so that parents and patients won't experience an acute and potentially anaphylactic reaction at home when trying a food for the first time. At Eden's annual five-year-old appointment, his blood-test results had declined to a low level for shrimp, crab, and lobster so challenges were considered because there was a chance that Eden was no longer allergic to those foods. But blood tests only measure the amount of allergic antibodies in the body. Test results can't predict with total accuracy whether a person would have an allergic reaction to a food or what symptoms would occur if the allergy still exists.

According to current NIH guidelines, food allergies should be diagnosed by employing a multifaceted approach that includes a detailed patient history, a diet diary, an elimination diet, skin tests, blood tests, and oral/food challenges. After years of studying Eden's blood tests, I've noticed that his results can fluctuate for no apparent reason. But as the numerical results (the test results are on a scale from .35 to 100) drop significantly, the food in question may become tolerable. Or it may not. Only Eden's body can know whether a food becomes tolerable. For example, a few years ago his egg result dropped, but not into the undetectable range. Since that time he can tolerate hardboiled eggs and some forms of extensively heated eggs but lesser versions cause his throat and mouth to itch to the point where he asks for Benadryl.

A few months before our seafood challenge, Doctor Anderson allowed me to choose one shellfish out of three possible choices: shrimp, lobster, and crab. I opted for shrimp.

"Very good," she affirmed. "Some of our children have done very well with shrimp in their diet."

There was a brief silence during which I thought, *Are you kidding me? Why didn't his numbers go lower for milk or egg or peas even? Kid food?* That was followed by more silence during which I created guilt-driven shrimp gratitude mantras. *Some kids must like shrimp and I just don't know them. It's a very good sign. What a nice protein source. Shrimp rocks.* Then we set the date.

A week after Eden graduated from preschool, I set my alarm for 6 a.m., pattered into my kitchen, and steamed about a half pound of organic peeled shrimp while sipping black tea and honey. Sometimes I order shellfish in restaurants, but I rarely cook it. Rarely meaning almost never. Rarely meaning I recoiled at the oceanic smell, pulled up the kitchen window, and risked the noise of the oven vent while I bathed the shrimp in ice. Then I packed it up along with a container of ketchup for Eden and two lemon wedges for me in case I needed to model my relish for his seafood breakfast. Then I added three books, a pack of gum (no food allowed except shrimp), and a few DVDs. The DVDs proved extraneous because the departmental pediatric allergy DVD player was broken that day. Thus the *SpongeBob* marathon.

But enough about life in Bikini Bottom. Eden went into his challenge with a positive attitude.

"What's it like?" he asked repeatedly on the way over.

"It's good. I really like shrimp."

"But what does it taste like?"

What does shrimp taste like? "Like something tasty," I answered.

After a brief chat with Doctor Anderson, a nurse set Eden in a chair with a timer by his side. "Let me know when this beeps if I'm not back here," she instructed me. Then she dived into my Tupperware with a plastic fork and knife, cutting furiously. "Here you go!" She held a forkful cheerily. To my surprise, Eden opened his mouth like a nesting baby bird. He chewed and chewed. I studied his face, arms, and legs while pretending to study the wall behind him. "Great," said the nurse. "How do you feel?"

"Great!" answered Eden.

"Then I'll be back!" And she was. About five more times in the course of one hour, each time spooning in one more bite and then checking Eden's pulse, breathing, and skin tone. Eden chewed and swallowed, and nothing allergic happened. Another three hours of observation and having no reaction, he rose to the challenge and emerged as a safe and unfettered shrimp eater. We walked the sunny streets home strangely proud.

Since then I've cooked shrimp for all of us a dozen times. I've grilled it on a barbecue, breaded and fried it, steamed and sautéed it. Drew and I have chomped shrimp with ravenous enthusiasm. The first time I made it for him, Eden ate one and a half shrimp and then stopped with the pronouncement, "It's kind of chewy. I'll stop now."

The second time, Eden took two bites. He has refused it since. Not surprisingly, Dayna declined every shrimp opportunity. And after some soul-searching I've decided it's fine that Eden doesn't want to eat shrimp. We all have foods that we can eat but don't like. Why would I impose a different ideology on him? Sure, I wonder how much of Eden's palate had been built by experiences such as food challenges, food reactions, fear, and denial versus sheer pleasure. I know other allergy parents who also become frustrated when their allergic child rejects their safe and nutritious food alternatives: the sunflower seed butter or soy butter meant to stand in for peanut butter or the calcium-fortified orange juice that Eden asserts is "acidy." (Why, oh why did I ever say that where he could hear me?) But like so many other parents, I'm trying to create a new normal—fresh rules for the familiar, and familiar rules for the unusual.

A perfectly normal day can easily and abruptly turn wrenching with the surprise of an allergic reaction. Once I watched a news show featuring parents of food-allergic children. One mother teared up as she concluded her interview: "It was just a morning like any other morning. And that one simple thing. Pouring the wrong milk. And the whole day was spent in the emergency room. Who could have known when we woke up that day?" She described my truth. Risks are deceptive: a tired lazy morning, the cartons next to each other on the shelf—food safety is so simple yet so fallible. As I'm writing this, an e-mail alert comes into my in-box informing me that a particular brand of breaded okra has just been recalled for "undeclared milk." I get these alerts daily: pastries with undeclared nuts, ice cream with undeclared wheat, fish sticks with undeclared egg. Although some of the alerts may seem silly to the nonallergic, they are one more reminder to keep the familiar in check in little ways, such as assigning Eden a distinct plate and a different spoon rest during family meal preparations so that I don't do that one simple thing wrong.

Our time with Eden has shown us that three-alarm days are in fact the exception to false-alarm days. But both are reminders that we live differently. Thankfully, I practice false alarms more often. I've learned that I'm going to have capricious moments of fear for as long as Eden has food allergies. Just a few months ago I got very scared in the middle of a salon appointment. I was getting a haircut because Dayna and Eden had one of those "why is school closed again?" days off, and so I had asked my father if he wanted to spend time with his grandkids. He did. The plan was for him to take both kids to the park for a picnic lunch while I went to get my neglected scraggly split ends trimmed. My father had taken the kids out like that many times.

The moment the front door clicked behind them, I began chucking things into my shoulder bag, calculating whether my appointment had opened a window of unexpected extra time. Minutes later, as I sat beneath the clicking metal blades, half listening to the stylist's chattered queries, I continued the estimations made by all mothers who rely on school hours and the kindness of extended family to accomplish more than is humanely possible. *If I go to the drugstore on the block, I can probably send that e-mail before they're back, and we have enough straws, so I can get tissues tonight. . . .* And then I remembered that I had meant to remind my father that the children's sandwiches were labeled with a *D* and an *E* in Sharpie pen on the outer foil, which was another precautionary habit of mine. *Did I remind him? Will he see those letters before Eden can take a bite? No way would they start eating that fast. Dayna's was cheese and mustard. Damn. Damn. No, he'll see it. Damn. He will.*

I didn't realize I was muttering my inner monologue out loud until my hairstylist poised her scissors over my head. "Everything okay?" I looked forward and saw my knotted brows in the mirror. For the first time in our three-year relationship my Goth, tattooed, pierced, twentysomething, Hello Kitty, hangover-sporting hairstylist blinked at me with genuine curiosity. In the reflection of her kohl-lined bloodshot eyes I saw all the other times I had silently (or not so silently) pantomimed my anxieties in public without seeing myself, and I wasn't a pretty sight.

One more moral of my haircut gone wild: emergency medication was invented for errors. Parents like me must build up enough faith to send our children out into the world as long as their emergency kits are there with them. My father had it with him that day, as should any caregiver of an allergic child. But yes, I've had other antics, such as exiting in the middle of gym class to phone home the crucial information that the pan on the stove may not have been run through the dishwasher and so could have some butter residue.

I'm going to guess that almost all parents think about the worst— the what if?—at least once in a while. And so I've even asked myself what would be worse—if Eden ate deadly food on my watch or, with good or careless intentions, on someone else's? Would it matter? My answer growls back at me with bared teeth for daring to ask: "No, no, no, you idiot! How could it matter whether you spend the rest of your life trying to forgive a friend or Drew or a stranger or yourself?" And still the same animal purrs into my ear in the dark hours: "Wait! Shhh. Now just think it. *Think it.*" And then I do. My sweet boy could in a moment be gone because and only because he opened his mouth to eat. How can I think it?

Our bulky kits of antihistamine and EpiPens must be with us because you never know. The odds are against disaster, yet the allergic types can defy them without warning. Again, people who have one type of allergy often are more likely to have other types of allergic problems. Just this past winter, Eden had a new allergic reaction. Yep. There we were in Central Park just like a hundred other days, when Eden turned to me and said, "Can we leave? I'm cold, and my face is so, so itchy!" I volunteered to take him home while Drew rallied on with Dayna. Not twenty feet later, hives began to spread across Eden's cheeks, which were turning red and puffy. "Owww! Now my face hurts."

My mind flashed back a few years to a support group meeting at which a mother had described this experience of "cold hives." I thought fast. Eden hadn't eaten anything new that day. He hadn't eaten for a few hours. I guessed that he must have cold hives like that other child. After I hustled out the Benadryl and hustled us home, the hives receded after the medicine had time to work in a warm bath. By the time Drew and Dayna burst in, snow dripping off their boots, I had stopped running through my mental packing list for the emergency room.

Eden's allergic reaction happened on a Saturday, so I had an indulgent day of Googling before speaking with his allergist, Doctor Anderson. I learned that cold-induced hives can appear as a one-time incident or, um, cold-induced urticaria can last a decade or more. After a brief phone call that Monday, I learned that I should keep him as unexposed as possible in low temperatures by dressing him warmly and covering his exposed skin with a barrier cream. I would of course continue to carry our emergency kit even when headed out for a wintertime errand.

New normal. What's really normal? Video games are in my parenting world. We have several Wii video games. In our collection of customizable Wii video characters, Dayna created one she named Doctor Jacobs, after our osteopath. Given the limits of technology, his dark beard and thick glasses bear an uncanny resemblance. What else? Well, Eden learned to read along with most of his classmates in kindergarten. But he can scan and interpret a food label with more comprehension than can children twice his age. Occasionally, I've heard Eden's encouraging "Here's your remedy, Spider-Man!" before he pours little paper balls over the poor action figure's face. That's right. In our normal, young children explain the difference between soy lecithin and soy protein, and yes, even superheroes can have food allergies.

Will Eden ever be able to eat like most other kids? Maybe. Maybe not. Looking at Eden now, at eight years old, I can understand why I'm repeatedly asked: "But he will outgrow it, right?" He looks and acts like a typical little boy, a boy who might outgrow things. This is Eden right now: He is very small with delicate facial bones. He is emotionally contained. He is learning to skateboard with Dayna but finds it tiring. It's easier to scoot around our neighborhood on his Razor scooter. He can't stop thinking about presents until he opens them. His favorite prebedtime series is *Diary of a Wimpy Kid,* but during the day he reads J. K. Rowling books and other children's fantasy novels and, like his sister, leaves piles of books in his wake. He takes guitar lessons but practices reluctantly. Sometimes he lets me beat him at UNO when he could easily take the win. His expression is usually thoughtful. Now and then he blinks back tears at silly disappointments, but when he is excited, he flashes a face-splitting grin. In school he likes math and figuring numbers in his head: "It's 143 days until my birthday." He plays handheld electronic games as if all life hinged on his score. And one evening when I asked him if he wanted a "special" side dish with hamburgers, he said, "Cotton candy is pretty special," with a lack of guile that made me giddy.

So maybe Eden will outgrow his allergies.

I have a recurring outgrowing-it fantasy. Eden and I sit at a low table, on soft pillows, legs crossed beneath us. Everyone we love is there, and in front of us there is a feast. There are fried wonton dumplings stuffed with juicy pork shards and small bowls of shiny soy sauce; rounds of garlic toast; slivers of roast beef; chicken mole and avocado inside wedges of tortilla; puff pastries stuffed with crumbly cheddar cheese and chives; chilled lump crabmeat with shallot cream; thin pizzas flecked with buffalo mozzarella and oregano; fried chicken legs circling twice-baked potatoes browned to soft peaks; Bibb lettuce dressed with radishes and ranch dressing; fluffy creamed spinach casseroles steaming from their middle; Caesar salads anointed with homemade garlic croutons; bowls of ropy pasta, yellow teardrop tomatoes, pesto, and walnuts; breaded lemon sole and Spanish rice; bite-sized ravioli.

For dessert there are tubs of ice cream. There is mint chip, chocolate, butter pecan, and cookies and cream; a gravy bowl of hot butterscotch and one of hot fudge; painted ceramic crockery piled with fresh strawberries and blueberries soaked in whipped cream; angel food cupcakes capped with bonnets of yellow frosting; lumpy peanut butter cookies with nubs of toasted peanuts sticking out; chocolate éclairs; and two pies, one lemon meringue with droplets of caramelized sugar beading off its top and the other coconut cream with a graham cracker crust. We all laugh and pass plates. Dayna trades a crunchy bit of pie crust for a dollop of Eden's melting whipped cream. Eden reaches, takes, and offers. Eden is the prince. I move his plate closer, butter his dinner roll. Our lips are anointed with oils. Eden has outgrown it. He rules our table.

Years back, outgrowing it usually came up during park bench conversations. There was that time my dentist required the outline of Eden's life's story for me to explain why, yes, he was a lousy sleeper, and yes, my sleep was frequently interrupted, and consequently why, possibly, I ground my teeth nocturnally. Now both children spend their days in school instead of at the playground. I spend my days writing the stories that tell themselves to me as I tell them. When I explain Eden for the first time, most people exclaim, "But he'll outgrow it!?" Because that is what should happen, yes? Eden and the other three million food-allergic children in the United States should outgrow their allergies. That seems like the right answer to all of us since our sisters, our cousins, and ourselves, we, they, outgrew allergies. The question isn't really a question; it is a kind of self-assurance hiding under the humility of its question mark. And there isn't, in fact, a clear and reassuring answer.

Unfortunately, most of today's children who have multiple life-threatening food allergies are too young to reveal what the statistics may show us over their lifetimes. What is known is that theirs is a new generation of food allergies. In 2007, a study from the specialty allergy clinic at John Hopkins Children's Center revealed that milk allergy persisted much longer in life than previously was assumed. Among 800 children with a milk allergy, only 19 percent had outgrown it by age four, though 79 percent had outgrown it by age sixteen. (Ouch. Those are prime years when children are at risk for inadequate calcium intake.) Similar trends were seen in studies on egg allergy outgrowth. Only 4 percent outgrew egg allergy by age four, 37 percent outgrew it by age ten, and 68 percent outgrew it by age sixteen.[23]

Furthermore, the Johns Hopkins Children's Center team found that in interpreting a child's blood levels of milk and egg IgE antibodies, the higher the level of antibodies was, the less likely it was that a child would outgrow the allergy soon. Eden's blood tests for milk, soy, tree nuts, peanuts, lentils, chickpeas, green peas, and sesame seeds have shown antibodies in an amount over 100 (on a scale from .35 to 100) for many years. I can still remember when Eden's first allergist told me that he had an unusually high histamine level. Now I understand the significance of that comment. And in light of that, I don't want Eden to become the muse for a sorry story, inspiring more of the tired expressions I've been offered: "God gives you what you can handle" and "It's always something." Those ideas might comfort other people, but I want a livable treatment or cure for my son.

Don't I care about the cause of Eden's allergies too? I do. I'd care a lot more if knowledge of the cause led researchers to a cure. Several years ago, I attended a public symposium at Mount Sinai Medical Center. The large auditorium was almost full. Two women sitting in front of me were commiserating: "Well, it's not like I can go anywhere without a kitchen. Remember Florida? What a disaster!" I pictured a minifridge with shelves an inch too small for fitting rice milk cartons, a breakfast buffet oozing with butter, beachside stands overrun with grilled calamari and cheeseburgers.

The first doctor to speak stepped up to the microphone and warned, "I'm taking you back to Biology 101!" He spoke about the current hygiene hypothesis and why it was becoming a popular explanation for the worldwide rise in allergies. Using an overhead projector, he drew a picture of an immune system with two arms. He explained that each arm was responsible for a different response: one arm was in charge of fighting bacteria and viruses, and the other arm primarily fought parasites. The parasite arm was the one responsible for classic allergic responses such as releasing histamines, mucus, and other chemical mediators.

Then the doctor stopped drawing and placed his marker on the podium for a moment. Facing us, he suggested that if a young immune system doesn't meet enough viruses and bacteria or doesn't meet the right kind, that response network may not be stimulated sufficiently. In response, the entire immune system might teeter off balance and overactivate the parasite-fighting response. This imbalance could have caused Eden's immune system to fight the wrong things—food proteins, pollens, animal dander—attacking them as it would an enemy.

The hygiene hypothesis is a popular theory for the increase in food allergies. In 2004, the National Institute of Allergy and Infectious Disease followed the medical records of 835 children from birth to age one, documenting any fever-related episodes. At six to seven years, more than half of the children were evaluated again for their sensitivity to common allergens such as dust mites, ragweed, and cats. Among the children who didn't experience a fever during their first year, 50 percent showed allergic sensitivity. Among those who had one fever, the percentage dropped to 46 percent. But among the children who had two or more fevers, only 31 percent showed allergic sensitivity.[24] So children might have fewer allergies if society allowed them to get dirtier and sicker?

But how much sicker? What about the advances modern medicine has made in eradicating childhood diseases such as polio? And how much dirtier? Do we want our children exposed to more parasites? The helminth hypothesis is nearly identical to the hygiene hypothesis but focuses exclusively on parasites. Helminths are worms that can invade a person's body and live in the intestinal tract. In the 1980s researchers studied the immune responses of Venezuelan Indians. They found that among those who lived in the rain forest and were heavily infected with worms, under 10 percent had allergies. But a whopping 43 percent of the wealthier Venezuelan Indians who lived in cities and were only lightly infected with worms had allergies.[25] A "worm versus wealth" theory is the yang to the yin of the hygiene hypothesis: maybe we need more exposure to parasites to balance our reduced exposure to bacteria and viruses. Either way, clean water and food, antibiotics, and reduced exposure to parasites, animals, viruses, and infectious diseases may have contributed to the increase in allergies worldwide.

But these ideas don't offer obvious solutions to parents. A few years ago, a well-known research immunologist infected himself with hookworm larvae and reduced his allergic symptoms. (Shudder.) There isn't evidence that an allergic kid like Eden would benefit from exposure to parasites or from an occasional lick of a New York City subway pole. (Dramatic shudder.) When people ask me why Eden has allergies and I answer, "Well, most doctors favor the hygiene hypothesis," their next question predictably has the phrase *antibacterial hand wipes* in it. How to segue toward the less inviting explanation, "Well, some scientists believe our world is too clean. . . ." Sure, I could then launch into a monologue about contaminated water except that my own kitchen counter is never without a full pitcher of filtered water with its reassuring filter-change-reminder sticker.

My friends are open to switching their hand soap to Burt's Bees All Natural but balk at the idea of unfiltered water and unwashed hands. I get it. I want to control my children's health too. I want to benefit from medical progress while circumventing nature's backlash. The hard truth is that if I had let Eden play in the mud like a baby farm animal, he still might have gotten allergies. No one has the answers, and these hypotheses are confounded by genetics and environment.

Other allergy ideas, though unproven, include the role of vaccines, genetic engineering of foods, and timing of food introduction. The increased pediatric vaccination schedule has been called out as a culprit in causing food allergies to increase. Perhaps vaccination has led to overstimulation of the immune system. Or are the vaccines protecting our children from the infections that may prevent allergies? Other voices speak out against our industrial and agricultural practices. Perhaps crossbreeding and genetic engineering are responsible for our children's toxic overload. Perhaps all those alterations to our food are creating new proteins that are being recognized by our IgE antibodies. Some parents, more afraid of human-made toxins than of germs or bacteria, ask me, "What about all those pesticides? I only buy organic. Don't you?" Well, no, not always. Or are we not exposing our children to foods at the right time in life— should it be earlier or later? Though I don't want to expose my children to the by-products of human industry, every factor from cooking methods, socioeconomic status, gender, and exposure to pool chlorine, fetal head size, early exposure to foods, late exposure to foods, and country of birth has been examined in terms of its contribution to food allergies. To which should I subscribe? Some of those circumstances have proved to be instrumental, but none have been proved to be the sole determining factor.

Meanwhile, I've listened to many mothers assume the burden of their children's allergies by citing their diet during pregnancy. Yet an expecting mother's diet hasn't been proved to cause her children's food allergies. We parents want to know why things happen to our children. We are ready to bear the guilt: *Bring it on! You can't handle the guilt! I can!* When Eden was born, he was given antibiotics to clear excess fluid from his lungs. The NICU (neonatal intensive care unit) staff advised us. They said so. Was that it? Did those antibiotics tip Eden's first domino?

And then there is guilt's evil twin, blame. In 2008, six years after my first pediatrician insisted that Eden wasn't reacting allergically to his milk-based formula, the American Academy of Pediatrics published a report that advised that for infants with Eden's health history the use of "an extensively hydrolyzed formula" might "delay or prevent atopic dermatitis.[26] Every time I think about that AAP report, I swallow a raw and unending frustration. Could I have slowed or prevented the allergic cascade? Was that it?

Then again, Eden was vaccinated on the recommended schedule while his food allergies were emerging. Was that it?

Maybe we think we gave our children the wrong food or too many antibiotics. Maybe we wake up in the middle of night wondering if we should have kept them away from the cats or the peanut proteins we leaked through our breast milk. Or we should have done the opposite. Maybe we did something bad that was supposed to be good for our children. But as the medical community looks for answers, I keep looking for ways to help Eden live well.

In Eden's case, his osteopath aims to cure him in time for college, as he did for his own son. I hope. We hope. Not to be saved but to work with Doctor Jacobs toward our goal by adhering to his recommendations, however unique. Conventional allergists and immunologists are focused on finding successful treatments for food allergies. They don't know whether those will turn out to be cures or regimens requiring ongoing administration. It's 2011 as I write this, and there are several promising treatments in progress that might help Eden and other children with food allergies.

Closest to my home, there is a pill undergoing trials that is composed of nine different botanical herbs. Its formula is based on a 2,000-year-old Chinese remedy. Peanut allergy is relatively rare in China, and the traditional herbal formula is based on an ancient formulation called Wu Mei Wan that was prescribed for colic, vomiting, chronic diarrhea, dysentery, or "collapse," and Lingzhi, which is known to have anti-inflammatory and antiallergy properties. Named FAHF-2, the initial safety study was completed and the second phase to determine efficacy is now in progress, with the goal that it be used as an herbal drug for allergies to peanuts, tree nuts, fish, and/or shellfish.

China is far from Manhattan, but it happens that the study, led by Doctor Xiu-Min Li, is being conducted at Mount Sinai Medical Center, where Eden is a patient.

I'm keeping abreast of two additional therapies currently undergoing clinical trials. These therapies could easily be confused since both involve ingesting a teeny-tiny bit of allergen. The first is Oral Immunotherapy (OIT). Oral Immunotherapy is conducted under strict medical supervision, and it involves patients swallowing very small amounts of the foods that trigger their allergies. We're talking nano small. The doses start at $\frac{1}{1000}$ of a peanut.

Duke and Arkansas Children's Hospital began enrolling patients in studies for OIT and published results in 2009. Of the 39 children participating in the study, 29 of 39 were able to complete the study and participated in oral food challenges to peanuts after 4 to 22 months of maintenance therapy. Overall, 27 of the 29 were able to tolerate the highest dose of peanut at the challenge, which indicated that they were successfully desensitized to peanut protein.[27]

The idea behind OIT is for children to build their immunity to the foods to which they are allergic, and it seems that some of the food-allergic children are showing positive immunologic changes in a fairly short period. It's not certain, though. Currently, because the pool of children who are eating peanuts at home and also are off treatment is so small, researchers can't say with absolute certainty that the success was due to OIT or that possibly those children outgrew their allergies in the meantime.

Next step for OIT is a blind study in which children on treatment are compared with an off-treatment placebo control group. At this point there are more questions than answers. For one thing, there are cautions about children who are too sensitive to peanuts undergoing OIT. Second, OIT studies involving milk and eggs just began alongside peanut OIT. A number of children probably will drop out because of side effects. Since these itty-bitty antiallergy drops are taken at home after a certain point of progression, no one knows if allergic reactions will occur as a result of changes in a child's daily physical state. For example, if a child has a head cold or has just exercised rigorously, he may have had an allergic reaction to the dose on that day but would be fine with the same dose had he not been sick or especially tired.

Our bodies aren't designed to heal big-picture problems while coping with smaller circumstantial distractions. It's common knowledge among parents of allergic children that you don't offer a child a new food if that child is even slightly sick or fatigued. The changing hormones of a growing body are another consideration. Oral Immunotherapy, if administered incorrectly, has the potential to cause a severe allergic reaction (including anaphylaxis) in a food-allergic child because of other variables.

The second allergy treatment is called sublingual immunotherapy (SLIT). There is actually a big difference between SLIT and OIT. Whereas Oral Immunotherapy involves swallowing a very small amount of an allergen in increasing amounts, SLIT involves a liquid or tablet of diluted allergen that is dissolved under the tongue. There are several problems with this as a treatment for food allergies. One is that studies involving SLIT as a remedy for environmental (not food) allergies haven't been consistently successful. Another is that some researchers believe there is a stronger possibility of an anaphylactic reaction in food-allergic children. Overall, less is known about SLIT in treating food allergies.

The last option I've considered as a possible future treatment for Eden is an injection that is already available for asthma sufferers under the trade name Xolair. It is also available in a generic form that is called omalizumab. Xolair is an anti-IgE medication. The drug attaches to IgE molecules in the bloodstream and it also causes mast cells to have fewer IgE antibodies on their surfaces; this prevents the mast cells from sending out the nasty little histamines that cause allergic reactions.

Xolair's history as a treatment for allergies is complicated and political. It got a delayed start years ago when competing pharmaceutical companies discovered they were both making an anti-IgE product. One of those products, talizumab, developed by Tanox, a Houston-based biopharmaceutical company, was fast-tracked by the FDA and the clinical trials, as described in the *New England Journal of Medicine*, went so well that one participant went from sensitivity at half a peanut to tolerating nine peanuts. The 2003 breakthrough prompted *Scientific American* to publish an article titled "New Drug May Mitigate Peanut Allergy."[28] Then two other drug companies, Genentech and Novartis, took Tanox to court, claiming that talizumab was too similar to their anti-IgE drug Xolair. The legal entanglement went on for years, and eventually the three companies formed a partnership agreement in which Xolair was chosen for its superior manufacturing process.

Currently, Xolair is approved for asthma treatment and is being retested in conjunction with Oral Immunotherapy for food allergies. Some studies suggested that milk-allergic children who had milk protein OIT became less sensitive in the short term but not the long term. Now Xolair is being tested in conjunction with OIT in an effort to decrease side effects related to OIT, increase OIT's protection against allergic reactions, and hopefully have longer-term effectiveness

I've witnessed Xolair's effect on asthma. My mother has had asthma for fifty years, and just a few years ago her pulmonologist offered her the option of a monthly Xolair injection. She was having more asthmatic flairs that required stronger and stronger medications. Her pulmonologist felt that a Xolair shot might enable her to reduce her medications along with her bouts of breathing distress. "Honey, I just want to be able to keep traveling, doing things," she confessed to me. "I don't want to feel afraid to go away." Knowing what that apprehension felt like, I didn't want it for her either.

I read about Xolair and helped my mother decide whether she wanted to try it. I learned that the risks were, in our opinion, minimal for a woman of her health and age and the potential gains were significant.

And they were. Within a few months of her monthly Xolair injection, my mother said she felt more energetic (asthma is tiring whether you are old or young), and she has safely reduced her daily medications.

So what if? So what if in the future Xolair is to be an effective treatment (either alone or in combination with OIT) for food allergies? Well, I've sat next to my mother while she's had her injection. The serum is thick. "It hurts," she admits. And here's my other concern: Ideally, I would like for Eden's body to learn how to be less allergic. I'd like his body to heal itself. And of course, all these solutions have question marks about long-term use. My mother is in her seventies. Eden is seven.

Maybe a treatment will come before we really need it. Studies have shown that teens are "more likely to engage in risk-taking behaviors when it comes to their food allergies." *The Journal of Allergy and Clinical Immunology* describes a study done on a large university campus that showed that only 39 percent of students with an identified allergy consistently avoided that allergen and only 47 percent of the students consistently carried their medications.[29] Some parents in my support group have described evidence of defiance or carelessness on the part of their children that resulted in emergency room visits.

It's maddening, though. Despite the justified concerns about keeping food-allergic children safe, that topic has an controversial history in parenting circles and the media. Questions have arisen about the accuracy of allergy tests, but parents rely on them to gauge their children's safety. These tests are all we have to order our lives around besides our children's allergic reactions. Other questions come from parents who believe that parents of food allergic children exaggerate the dangers. Sometimes it seems that the nonallergic world is waiting for better proof of our experience.

I have my own theories about this allergic cynicism. Some parents may believe in life-threatening food allergies, but they want to control what they and their children eat. Those people interpret a restriction, such as a nut-free school, as an assault on their autonomy. Maybe these naysayers are simply protecting the right to eat freely. Maybe they are disturbed by the idea that they or their children may be denied a food. Was there plain primal instinct at play when a parent said to me, "No way would I be okay if we couldn't pack Robert's peanut butter and jelly lunch! It's the only sandwich he'll eat." Do parents with ample means to feed their children nevertheless fear their children's hunger?

When it comes to food allergy protocol, I try to see any negativity as emotional, not thoughtless or obstinate. I once met a woman on the beach whose child was born with a cleft palate. When we discussed our children, she repeated her pastor's words to me: "What people do not understand, they reject." I was looking at Eden while she spoke. He was glowingly tan, scooping energetically into the sand. He did not look like a child who needed accommodating. Food allergies are like that. They are invisible until they attack.

I want to believe that our communities can come to a reasonable and peaceful consensus regarding our children's food allergies, with any food restrictions thoughtfully tailored to each community. I think that the general population and those in schools shouldn't be limited more than is medically necessary but enough to ensure the maximum safety for the maximum amount of children. I feel that peanut-free classrooms might be applicable to younger children who eat with their hands and share toys but that those restrictions may backfire for many reasons in older populations.

My measures to teach Eden how to keep himself safe are based on the assumption that he will be in situations where he is not safe. I've learned these measures from my fellow food allergy parents. Research continues to illustrate his challenging reality. When there is a chink in our children's armor, maybe an uncompromising school administrator or an uninformed camp counselor, the strongholds fold inward and topple upon the whole family. Not surprisingly, children can misunderstand their food-allergic classmates. A 2001 National Institute of Child Health and Human

Development study found that about 17 percent of children in grades six to ten reported being bullied. By comparison, 50 percent of kids in that age group in the food allergy study were reported to have experienced bullying, teasing, or harassment.[30]

Most parents who have allergic children are focused on getting through each day. We aren't derailed by controversy, only by our children's well-being. Folding a chronic and potentially deadly health issue into each moment is less effort for our young. For us, it is work. We are busy. We are baking, freezing quantities of cupcakes, stowing spare nebulizers in our cars, training grandparents to jab needles into their grandchildren's thighs, duplicating forms and prescriptions, organizing kitchen shelves, talking to our children about their choices and their disappointments, preparing for certain holidays weeks ahead, and trying all the while to believe that it won't always be like this. Some parents find an outlet in speaking out, publicizing the issues, forwarding petitions for improved food allergy laws. Some provide resources or products to parents like themselves. I don't know how I would manage if I didn't write my stories.

I think Eden and Dayna have been encouraged by my openness. Eden retells his stories: a memorable reaction or a time he reminded me to read the label. These descriptions are seamlessly woven into the lore of our family along with more typical occasions such as fall apple picking, annual celebrations, and silly moments in the car. Children don't need to know more than they need. Both of our children are somewhat talented worriers, and so I try to interject humor, silly phrases, and jokes in various versions of our allergy stories and allergy planning. And when I catch Eden adopting my tone, riffing back at me when I make a small mistake—"Umm, Mom, no offense, but you gave me the wrong dessert. Mom? Uhhh, Nestlé *Crunch* Bites? No offense, but that's Dayna's. Can I have *my* chocolate chips, puh-lease?"—I believe I'm getting it right.

Still, both children understand that food allergies have made our life different. The other night for dinner we shared a pot of spaghetti doused with olive oil. I chopped tomatoes and olives into a bottled red sauce. Eden prefers his squirt of ketchup since fresh garlic sometimes still makes his mouth itch. I washed lettuce leaves and chopped cucumber since we dress our salads individually. Protein has become another issue. Drew recently gave up meat for health goals, and I joined him. Of course now, after her earlier vegetarian leanings, Dayna has decided she likes particular forms of red meat, whereas Eden prefers ground beef or chicken burgers. So we all had burgers—veggie, beef, and chicken, respectively. I know there are other families that eat in a similar Rubik's Cube fashion despite the trendy call for a home-cooked, local, sustainable, socially aware family dinner hour. But our menu originates from the necessity of the life and death category. Our plates are usually filled with subsets of our whole. New normal.

We have refashioned much of our lives. But we have what we need. In fact, we have so much. I've written an entire book about Eden's allergies while resisting the urge to describe why the softest, most velvety place in the world happens to be on the back of his neck. That is the spot I was stroking that day last summer just before Eden took his turn on one of those giant water slides, the kind that slosh and spin children in wild downward spirals and dump them screaming into pools. I waited for him at the bottom of the slide when snap, clap, the sun emerged from behind a cloud to halo the wet tangle of arms and legs that burst out of the water slide, more muskrat than child. Eden flew to me, screaming with rightful joy. After the waves of yellow shimmer and sound settled into a background of other children's voices, a patch of my heart remained warm and breathless from dancing with itself. Those days everything is exactly as it should be.

APPENDIX:
YOUR FAMILY'S LIFE WITH
FOOD ALLERGIES

THERE ARE MANY FOOD ALLERGY RESOURCES. There are books, organizations, and websites where you can find creative solutions and strategies to build a full and satisfying food-allergic life. The following suggestions are limited to my personal experiences and choices.

SEARCHING FOR A SAVIOR

Even with Doctor Anderson's help, I would make mistakes. She wasn't a deity, but she was a good partner for all of us.

Finding the right doctor to treat your child's food allergies is the first step in managing this chronic condition. Maybe you already have the right doctors and haven't had to look far. But if you don't believe that you and your child's needs are being taken care of by your current doctors, the first question you may ask yourself is, "Why?"

Here's a checklist of some possible answers:

- My doctor and I don't communicate well.
- I'm not comfortable with my doctor's diagnosis or treatment.
- The office is difficult for me to navigate (too busy, wrong hours, poor location, carelessness with paperwork).

Each of these answers may lead to more questions:

My doctor and I don't communicate well. Where do you think the lack of communication comes from? If you think your doctor is qualified, you should ask yourself how prepared you are for appointments. Writing your own notes and questions is crucial. I'll never forget the amount of time Drew and I spent putting together Eden's health history along with filling out the required hospital forms. I think of it as Eden's first story. Nevertheless, the time was well spent. I was too anxious at Eden's appointments to speak as clearly and calmly as I can now, and trying to remember so many details only adds to the anxiety. Anxiety leads to distraction, and distraction makes it really hard to hear anything.

I'm not comfortable with my doctor's diagnosis or treatment. What kind of doctor does your food-allergic child need? Some pediatricians handle food allergies knowledgably, especially if a child has a singular allergy, such as peanuts. If you feel that your diagnosis or treatment isn't correct or complete, you may want to consider a pediatric allergist in addition to a pediatrician. Or, you may be more concerned about your child's asthma than about his or her food allergies and prefer to see a pediatric pulmonologist and a pediatrician. Different combinations work for different children. If you can, get referrals from people you trust: your pediatrician or your friends. If you need more sources, visit these websites:

American Academy of Allergy, Asthma & Immunology (www.aaaai.org)
American College of Asthma, Allergy and Immunology (www.acaai.org)
American Medical Association (www.ama-asssn.org)

The doctor's office is difficult for me to navigate. Which aspects of the office make you uncomfortable? Eden's first pediatrician had a bustling practice. His second pediatrician practiced with two other partners, and I couldn't be certain which doctor we would see at appointments. That policy wasn't right for Eden. At that time, I felt he needed better continuity in his care. Currently, Eden sees a pediatric allergist at Mount Sinai, which is a large hospital. We balance that care by using a pediatrician (and an osteopath) who practice individually and can be reached after office hours. Of course there can be other policy issues, such as office hours or location, that have to be assessed as well.

A TABLE FOR FOUR

Meal planning is getting tricky.

When Eden was first diagnosed, meal planning was more than tricky. For me, parallel parking on Manhattan streets is tricky. Cooking for a child with food allergies is *very* hard. If you were like me before your child was diagnosed—the kind of parent who didn't feel all that comfortable in the kitchen, relied on shortcuts, or simply was not interested in cooking—adjusting to home-cooking all your child's meals is challenging. *What, no frozen organic chicken nuggets?*

Some mealtime advice:

Don't assume you can invent your own recipes right away.

Maybe you are a skilled cook, or maybe your child is allergic to a single ingredient. But if your child is allergic to multiple foods, simply omitting the allergic foods from normal recipes may result in crumbly meatballs and soggy cookies. I have a friend who has worked as a professional chef, and even she admits that she wouldn't know how to cook for Eden without a lot of trial and error.

Yet parents need to get food on the family table. In fact, Dayna and Eden often ask, "What's for dinner, Mom?" as early as breakfast time. You can begin with a cookbook created for people with allergies and eventually tweak the recipes to your liking. Be careful when attempting to make an allergen-free recipe "healthier." Many recipes, especially those for allergen-free baked goods, are carefully constructed to create a texture similar to that of the original recipe. For example, if you substitute honey for sugar, it could make for an soggy egg-free cake. You might want to start by looking through a variety of cookbooks that suit your child's allergic needs and your culinary style. You might want to emphasize organic whole grains or might want recipes that resemble ethnic or classic home-style meals. Many food allergy websites and blogs have recipes.

In addition to using cookbooks, I found it was very helpful to educate myself by reading books about food. The following books helped me plan my food shopping and family menus and nourish Eden despite his dietary restrictions.

The New Whole Foods Encyclopedia by Rebecca Wood

Don't be put off by the references to Ayurveda and Chinese medicine if you're not interested in that sort of thing. This book helped me answer many of my food-related questions. I learned how and why dried fruit gets sulfured, why a water chestnut isn't a nut but a chestnut is, and the difference between palm oil and palm kernel oil (trust me, huge difference). Another example: one of Eden's favorite "free-from" snacks is a dairy-free mock cheese doodle. It is dusted with "nutritional yeast," a substance I had never heard of, but after referencing this book, I learned it was safe for him.

Dictionary of Food Ingredients by Robert S. Igoe and Y. H. Hui

Anyone concerned about food allergies reads packaging labels over and over. Food labeling has become a new genre of reading in my household, but we do come across unrecognizable words. Do you know what alginic acid is? Where annatto coloring comes from? The Dictionary of Food Ingredients defines and offers derivations for all the ingredients that aren't recognizable as food, including those which are. This kind of reference volume can help you decide whether to purchase that dairy- and soy-free ice cream and offers information about foods you might have passed up.

On Food and Cooking: The Science and Lore of the Kitchen by Harold McGee

This is a dense book filled with more information about food and cooking than you may ever use. Assuming you've never been to culinary school, it can substitute as a crash course in the principles of baking (Why do we knead, and why is it bad to knead for too long?) and cooking (What's braising, and what's stewing?). It is technical and includes pictures of molecular food chains and graphs of the protein content in various flours. I doubt you will utilize the entire book unless you plan on doing your own milling and pickling. But I learned why pie crust is better when made with solid, not liquid, fat and why too much baking soda can make dough taste acidic and extra cooking water makes vegetables cook better but leaches their vitamins. The more I understand food, the more I understand how to keep Eden's food choices safe.

The recipe for my chocolate cake is from *The Food Allergy News Cookbook* (available on Amazon) and is called Ho Ho Sheet Cake. It's pretty simple. The recipe was developed during World War I, when butter, milk, and eggs were in short supply. I customized my Ho Ho Cake.

EDEN'S CHOCOLATE CAKE

3 CUPS FLOUR

2 CUPS SUGAR

2 TEASPOONS BAKING SODA

2/3 CUP UNSWEETENED COCOA POWDER (READ LABEL CAREFULLY BECAUSE SOME COCOA POWDERS ARE MADE ON EQUIPMENT WITH NUTS, ETC.)

2/3 CUP OIL *

2 CUPS PLUS 2 TEASPOONS WATER

2 TEASPOONS VANILLA EXTRACT

2 TEASPOONS POWDERED LEMON PEEL

2 TEASPOONS VINEGAR**

You can use any kind of safe vegetable oil or margarine. I think cakes taste richer when I use refined coconut oil or palm oil. If you are using a solid, liquefy it before adding, but I've used our countertop extra virgin olive oil in a time crunch and the cake still tasted yummy.

**Any kind will do, but I like to use white or dark balsamic vinegar.*

Preheat oven to 350 degrees. Grease a 9- by13-inch pan. Mix the dry ingredients first, using a fork to integrate the cocoa powder throughout. Add the oil and then the water. Add the vinegar last. The purpose of the vinegar is to "aerate" the batter. That means the vinegar creates air bubbles, which make the cake fluffy without eggs.

If you have an electric beater, use it. If you don't have one, consider buying one. I didn't have an electric beater before Eden was diagnosed, but I found that when baking without certain ingredients, such as eggs, I might need to manipulate food to get the right textures. Also, I like to make extralarge quantities of baked goods to freeze for unpredictable moments. An electric beater will save your arms from aching.

If you prefer to start baking with mixes, there are many packaged allergen-free mixes. In the years since Eden was diagnosed, there has been an explosion in free-from products. Like cookbooks, these mixes and products cater to different combinations of food allergies and other personal preferences.

A Word of Caution

In 2004 the total free-from food market was estimated to be a $1 billion business. Current estimates are at $4 billion, and the size of the industry is predicted to double over the next ten years. Beware of this bounty. You should read the labels of these products with as much scrutiny as you apply to mass-market fare. Why? First, food specialty items can be run on small production lines, which can allow for more shared equipment. Second, you should habitually read every label and call the manufacturers when in doubt.

What if certain foods are too difficult to replicate and share as a family? Rather than allow myself to feel deprived, I eat some of my favorite foods outside my home. Go out to dinner with your spouse or a friend or enjoy a buttery sugar cookie on a coffee break during your child's school day (and then wash your hands). Your allergic child will benefit from a parent who enjoys all of his or her food. **What if your allergic child has nonallergic siblings?** Those situations can be very conflicted. As the parents of two, we don't want Eden's sister, Dayna, to be denied the foods she likes or needs for nutritional reasons. In my experience, most parents end up striking their own bargains and balances among siblings. Some families take siblings out of the home for treats; others have a separate but equal policy; and still others, like mine, do a little of both. Also, anticipating situations that might seem unfair and talking about them in advance helps both children. For example, Dayna loves a particular dessert at our standby Italian restaurant, but there aren't any safe desserts there for Eden. When we go to that restaurant, we anticipate issues such as dessert. Sometimes we tote a safe dessert for Eden, but generally we all have dessert at home.

Other strategies I've used. Safe potato chips can be a good portable substitute when a nonallergic sibling wants to order French fries. Safe breadsticks are a good substitute when there will be a bread basket at a restaurant. There are going to be times your sibling policy gets stretched thin as a result of unexpected circumstances. That's when you might need to offer your allergic child an IOU. And just to reinforce the idea that food is not love, I often include a non-food-related bonus with my promise: "How about next time we go to a movie, you get to pick the one we see?"

RESCUING BUTTERFLIES

Is it that Eden won't *let you put him down or that you sense that he* can't *let you put him down? Is he controlling you or his needs?*

When my pediatrician first asked me that question, I wasn't sure how to answer, but I knew something was wrong. If you suspect that your food-allergic baby or child is having sensory issues (feeding issues are the most common ones), you shouldn't hesitate to call your pediatrician and begin asking questions.

Congress created what is known as Early Intervention in 1986. Early Intervention is designed to provide a range of services for children with disabilities under the age of three and their families. Don't be scared of the word *disability*. A disability can indicate a temporary delay in childhood development as well as a long-term delay. Each state establishes criteria for eligibility, and so available services vary on a state-by-state basis. Early Intervention really refers to a range of services designed for intervention at the early stages of an infant or toddler's disability. Infants or toddlers with disabilities in one or more of the following areas of development may qualify for Early Intervention: physical, cognitive, adaptive, communicative, and social and/or emotional development.

Early Intervention services include screening and assessment; family training, counseling, and home visits; speech therapy; occupational therapy; psychological services; audiology services; vision services; social work services; and transportation. These services are provided, with some exceptions, at no cost to the family.

EARLY INTERVENTION RESOURCES

For information about Early Intervention state by state, you can visit the National Early Childhood Technical Assistance Center's State Part C Coordinator Contact Listing

I found Team Eden only after moving Eden's case to a second social service agency. Agencies can have different therapists on staff and different protocols. For example, our first agency didn't have an available feeding therapist and offered me an occupational therapist as a substitute. The second agency appointed a feeding therapist who was also an occupational therapist. She was better for Eden. Also, the first agency required that Eden's physical therapy take place in its own outside facility, which was a very long subway ride from our home. The trip exhausted both of us. But our second agency sent our physical therapist to meet us at appropriate places nearby or in my home.

Again, agencies and other options can vary between states. The process and the paperwork involved can feel overwhelming, especially if you're simultaneously coping with your child's medical condition. Also, I found the evaluations emotionally draining. But if your child truly needs those therapies, I don't think you will have any regrets about the EI qualification process.

SWORD FIGHTING TO MUZAK

Despite more than a year of chronically interrupted sleep,
I had tapped into an endless supply of adrenaline that would fuel
our allergic new life.

If your young child has food allergies, sometimes you will have to be a warrior parent. You definitely will need to know more and do more to keep your child safe. Sometimes it will feel like you are running a marathon every day. But you can put down your coffee cup (or soda/chocolate bar/energy drink) once in a while. You don't need to reinvent the wheel.

New labeling laws require more ingredient information, but serving and production equipment can still be cross-contaminated. For example, I will buy Eden a safe sorbet scooped in an ice-cream store, but only if I watch the server use a freshly washed scooper. Drew forgot to make that request just once, and sure enough, Eden's throat started to itch after a few licks. Another example of hidden allergens surfaces in food production. We all develop our own rules: Some parents won't use food made "in the same factory" as an allergen. I might, but only if I have called and confirmed that the product isn't made on "shared equipment." Also, ingredients can change—another reason to read the label every time. A few months ago one of Eden's bread manufacturers changed its ingredients to include soy flour.

Maybe you have a good handle on the food but not on your feelings. Maybe, like me, you felt strangely isolated—as if having a kid with food allergies separated you from the world or, worse, from yourself. Maybe you feel like it happened to someone else or you would rather be someone else. Maybe you aren't sure how to speak to your allergic child or other children. Maybe you and your husband feel divided by the responsibility and mistrustful of each other. In my support group, I've learned that raising a child with food allergies can be like walking through a minefield. Different bombs explode for every family.

My therapist, Doctor Reiss, gave me a great deal of relief in a very short period because she was experienced in my issue and understood that I was there to solve specific problems and reduce a specific kind of anxiety. Parents everywhere go to battle for their children every day, and if you think you need professional help to manage your anxiety, you can seek out your own referral or check out the following organizations:

American Psychological Association (www.apa.org)

American Psychiatric Association (www.psych.org)

National Association of Social Workers (www.socialworkers.org)

FEEL HER BEATING

Most mothers keep watch;
our children's dangers are ships on the horizon.

If you're keeping watch and you see that your nonallergic child is signaling for help, obviously you'll want to solve his or her problems. Maybe your child feels that some of the food allergy restrictions and routines are unfair to him or her, or maybe, like my daughter, Dayna, your child is behaving differently toward food. What then? I tried to help my daughter regain her enthusiastic appetite in some usual and unusual ways. In addition to calling my pediatrician and our family therapist, I called an energy healer from New Mexico. That probably sounds like a weird choice, but I don't look back at my former self and chide that mother for her dramatics or weirdness. Calling an energy healer helped me as much as it may have helped Dayna (or maybe that's why it helped Dayna). I was comforted by the feeling that I was doing all I could to help both of my children. Don't worry about what your problem solving looks like. You may turn to family, a religious figure, an alternative healer, or a doctor for advice. The only disservice to your nonallergic child is to deny or delay his or her needs.

MEDICINE MOM

We parents can't make magic, but with our touches, our words,
and our love we can help our children find their medicine.
We can help them save themselves.

Every family has its own prescriptions for health. Some of my friends would never feel comfortable taking their children to an osteopathic doctor, as I do. I have friends who feed their children raw, unpasteurized milk and others who panic at the very thought of running out of frozen bagel bites. Some mothers rub Anbesol on their babies' sore gums, others use herbal gels, and others swear by whiskey. As I described in Chapter 1, "Searching for a Savior," parents must find the best medical care for their needs. But we all have to find doctors and medicine that will make our families' lives livable.

If you want to know more about the medical options that work for my family, here are some resources:

Osteopathy—There are over 50,000 osteopathic physicians and twenty accredited osteopathic medical colleges in the United States. For more information about the osteopathic profession, visit the website of the American Osteopathic Association (www.osteopathic.org)

If you want to know more about homeopathy, I like these books:

Everybody's Guide to Homeopathic Medicines by Stephen Cummings, MD, and Dana Ullman, MPH

The Consumer's Guide to Homeopathy by Dana Ullman, MPH

OPPOSITE DAY

I thought about how motherhood had reinvented my idols.
There was a time when rock stars were my rock stars.

If you feel that parenting has been life-changing, parenting a child with a health issue is even more transformative. Maybe you don't know how you feel about your new identity. Maybe you don't want to think of yourself as an allergy parent any more than you want your child to be an allergy kid. That's how I felt until I realized that I had to embrace a new life that would, for now, wind its way around the challenges of food allergies.

You may want to find a support group. The thought of joining anything and having to talk to strangers can be especially daunting if your child is newly diagnosed, but nothing can replace the perspectives of parents who already have experienced some of your challenges. Sure, I don't come home from every meeting and think, *well, thank God I didn't miss that one!* But I always gain from the reminder that there are parents out there doing what I do every single day.

To find a food allergy support group, check out the following:

- The Food Allergy & Anaphylaxis Network has a support group search tool that enables parents to look for a group in each state and city.
- The Food Allergy Initiative has a list of current groups around the world and a phone number if you can't find one in your area.
- You can ask your child's pediatrician or allergist.

Even with a baseline of information and support, it's easy to become stymied by the challenges of raising a food-allergic child. That's one reason I wrote a book about it.

NEW NORMAL

So maybe Eden will outgrow his allergies.

With the right treatments or cure, someday allergies may be a condition of the past. But in the meantime, we all have to create our new normal. We must continue to educate ourselves and those around us. Two organizations are indispensable resources: the Food Allergy & Anaphylaxis Network and the Food Allergy Initiative.

The Food Allergy & Anaphylaxis Network (FAAN)
www.foodallergy.org

This is the mission and history of FAAN as described on its website: "The Food Allergy and Anaphylaxis Network (FAAN) was established in 1991. FAAN's membership now stands at approximately 25,000 worldwide and includes families, dieticians, nurses, physicians, school staff, and representatives from government agencies and the food and pharmaceutical industries. FAAN serves as the communication link between the patient and others."

There is so much food allergy information on the FAAN website that I keep the site bookmarked on my computer's browser. FAAN is a one-stop shop for my questions on recent food allergy research, recalls, and updates. The website has food allergy information sheets, brochures, checklists, pamphlets, posters, presentations, and action plans (in many languages) for managing food allergies that you can download and give to caregivers, school personnel, and family members. The materials are insightful and concise.

For example, two of my favorite places on the FAAN website: The first is an animated explanation of how a reaction occurs, which helps you really see what is happening in your child's body. The second explains "How a Child Might Describe a Reaction." Like "That is too spicy!!" or "There's something stuck in my throat!" I showed both of those sections to Eden's grandparents so they could better recognize his reactions.

Now I remember that when my first allergist suggested I join FAAN and check out the website, I answered, "Sure, sure" with sincere intentions. But right after diagnoses, I felt too overwhelmed to read through the FAAN information. It felt like there were peanuts rattling in my head. Then, when I was ready to absorb them, reading materials about food allergies helped me feel less helpless and isolated.

Some things I got when I joined FAAN:

- *Food Allergy News:* a twelve-page bimonthly newsletter with strategies for managing food allergies, allergen-free recipes, and updates on food allergy research and legislative efforts.
- *Food Allergy News for Kids:* a newsletter written for children. (Eden likes reading which foods other kids are allergic to.)
- Discounted registration fee for the annual food allergy conferences.
- Special allergy alerts: These are notices of mislabeled and recalled food or pharmaceutical products, as well as advance notice of ingredient changes from some food manufacturers.

Food Allergy Initiative (FAI)
www.faiusa.org

Food Allergy Initiative was founded in 1998; its goal is to "fund research that seeks a cure; to improve diagnosis and treatment; and to keep patients safe through education and advocacy." The FAI website is filled with information, resources, online food allergy tools and applications, product information, and legislative information.

It's nice to have a printed book as well as online information. The handbook I used was *The Parent's Guide to Food Allergies* by Marianne S. Barber. It was one of the first handbooks of its kind, and I like the author's reasonable tone, simple format, and lengthy section titled "Coping." But it was written in 2001, and so a few of her views may be outdated.

Other popular food allergy handbooks include the following:

Flourishing with Food Allergies by A. Anderson
*How to Manage Your Child's Life-Threatening Food Allergies: Practical
    Tips for Everyday Life* by Linda Marienhoff Coss
Understanding Your Child's Food Allergies by Scott H. Sicherer
Food Allergies for Dummies by Robert A. Wood, MD
Asthma Allergies Children: A Parent's Guide by Dr. Paul Ehrlich, Dr.
    Larry Chiaramonte, and Henry Ehrlich

The winding road includes parties, restaurants, travel, camp, school—all the places and situations that aren't home. As I said, you don't have to reinvent the wheel, but you'll probably want to customize it. Here are some general resources:

Allergic Living magazine
888–881–7747
www.allergicliving.com

The American Academy of Allergy Asthma & Immunology
414–272–6071
800–822–2762
www.aaaai.org

Asthma and Allergy Foundation of America
800–7-ASTHMA
www.aafa.org

Asthma Allergies Children: A Parent's (Web) Guide
www.asthmaallergieschildren.com

Allergy & Asthma Network/Mothers of Asthmatics, Inc.
703–385–4403
800–878–4403
www.aanma.org

MedicAlert Foundation
888–633–4298
www.medicalert.org

Food Facts: Find Out What's Really In Your Food
www.foodfacts.com

Kids with Food Allergies Foundation
215–230–5394
www.kidswithfoodallergies.org

MOCHA (Mothers of Children Having Allergies)
www.mochallergies.org

ENDNOTES

1. "Allergy Facts and Figures," Asthma and Allergy Foundation of America, accessed March 28, 2011, http://www.aafa.org/display.cfm?id=9&sub=30.

2. "Infant Acid Reflux," Mayo Clinic, accessed March 30, 2011, http://www.mayoclinic.com/health/infant-acid-reflux/DS00787.

3. "Use of Hypoallergenic Infant Formulas," Maine Center for Disease Control & Prevention, Division of Family Health, accessed July 27, 2011, http://www.maine.gov/dhhs/wic/health/allergies.shtml

4. "Food Allergy Facts and Statistics," Food Allergy and Anaphylaxis Network (FAAN), accessed March 30, 2011, http://www.foodallergy.org/page/facts-and-stats.

5. "Diseases 101" (asthma and allergy statistics), American Academy of Allergy, Asthma & Immunology (AAAI), accessed March 30, 2011, http://www.aaaai.org/patients/gallery/prevention.asp?item=1a.

6. "Diseases 101," American Academy of Allergy, Asthma & Immunology.

7. "Milk and Egg Allergies Harder to Outgrow," *ScienceDaily*, December 17, 2007, http://www.sciencedaily.com/releases/2007/12/071215205437.htm.

8. "Severe Eczema Linked to Lasting Milk, Egg Allergy in Kids," *Bloomberg Businessweek*, March 21, 2011, http://www .businessweek.com/lifestyle/content/healthday/650899.html.

9. "Allergy Facts and Figures," Asthma and Allergy Foundation of America.

10. Annie Murphy Paul, "The First Ache," *New York Times*, February 10, 2008, http://www.nytimes.com/2008/02/10 /magazine/10Fetal-t.html?pagewanted=1&_r=1.

11. Mary E. Bollinger, Lynnda M. Dahlquist, Kim Mudd, Claire Sonntag, Lindsay Dillinger, and Kristine McKenna, "The Impact of Food Allergy on the Daily Activities of Children and Their Families," *Annals of Allergy, Asthma & Immunology*, March 2006, 96(3): 415–431, http://www.annallergy.org/article /S1081–1206(10)60908–8/abstract.

12. "FAI Study Examines Caregivers' Quality of Life," Food Allergy Initiative, accessed April 14, 2011, http://www.faiusa.org/page .aspx?pid=491

13. Adelle Davis, *Let's Have Healthy Children*, New York: Harcourt, Brace & World, 1959, p. 229.

14. Davis, *Let's Have Healthy Children*, p. 240.

15. K. Moore, T. J. David, C. S. Murray, F. Child, and P. D. Arkwright, "Effect of Childhood Eczema and Asthma on Parental Sleep and Well-Being: A Prospective Comparative Study," *British Journal of Dermatology*, March 2006, 154(3): 514–518, available at Wiley Online Library, http://onlinelibrary .wiley.com/doi/10.1111/j.1365-2133.2005.07082.x/abstract ;jsessionid=80687225A6B1A42B386E2BC056B1BC51.d02t02.

16. "Does the Atopic March Occur Equally in Both Genders?" American Academy of Allergy, Asthma & Immunology, May 21, 2008, http://www.aaaai.org/patients/jaci/2008archive/genders.asp.

17. J. M. Spergel and A. S. Paller, "Atopic Dermatitis and the Atopic March," *Journal of Allergy and Clinical Immunology*, December 2003, 112(6 Suppl): S118–127, citing earlier Swedish studies.

18. Amy M. Branum and Susan L. Lukacs, "Food Allergy among U.S. Children: Trends in Prevalence and Hospitalizations," National Center for Health Statistics (NCHS) Data Brief, No. 10, October 2008, http://www.cdc.gov/nchs/data/databriefs/db10.pdf.

19. "NIH-Funded Study Finds 2.5 Percent of Americans Have a Food Allergy," Occupational Health & Safety, accessed April 15, 2011, http://www.ohsonline.com/articles/2010/10/17/nih-funded-study-finds-25-percent-of-americans-have-a-food-allergy.aspx.

20. Tom Christopher, "Can Weeds Help Solve the Climate Crisis?" New York Times, June 29, 2008, http://www.nytimes.com/2008/06/29/magazine/29weeds-t.html.

21. Kanoko Matsuyama, "Japan's Post-War Cedar Trees Bring Allergy Misery (Update 1)," Bloomberg, April 2, 2008, http://www.bloomberg.com/apps/news?pid=newsarchive&sid=awYfpiU8JZJ4.

22. "Allergy Facts and Figures," Asthma and Allergy Foundation of America.

23. "Milk and Egg Allergies Harder to Outgrow," ScienceDaily.

24. "Early Fevers Associated with Lower Allergy Risk Later in Childhood," ScienceDaily, February 10, 2004, http://www.sciencedaily.com/releases/2004/02/040210080041.htm.

25. N. R. Lynch, R. López, G. Istúriz, and E. Tenías-Salazar, "Allergic Reactivity and Helminthic Infection in Amerindians of the Amazon Basin," International Archives of Allergy & Applied Immunology, 1983, 72(4): 369–372, in PubMed.gov (U.S. National Library of Medicine, National Institutes of Health), accessed April 16, 2011, http://www.ncbi.nlm.nih.gov/pubmed/6642708.

26. "Use of Hypoallergenic Infant Formulas," Maine Center for Disease Control & Prevention.

27. S. M. Jones, L. Pons. J. L. Roberts, et al., "Clinical Efficacy and Immune Regulation with Peanut Oral Immunotherapy," Journal of Allergy and Clinical Immunology, August 2009, 124(2):

292–300, 300.e1–97, in PubMed.gov (U.S. National Library of Medicine, National Institutes of Health), accessed August 1, 2011, http://www.ncbi.nlm.nih.gov/pubmed/19577283.

28. Sarah Graham, "New Drug May Mitigate Peanut Allergy," *Scientific American*, March 12, 2003, http://www.scientificamerican.com /article.cfm?id=new-drug-may-mitigate-pea.

29. Matthew J. Greenhawt, Andrew M. Singer, and Alan P. Baptist, "Food Allergy and Food Allergy among College Students," *Journal of Allergy and Clinical Immunology*, August 2009, 124(2):323–327, http://www.jacionline.org /article./50091-6749(09)00839-2/fulltext.

30. Bollinger et al., "The Impact of Food Allergy."

31. Elizabeth Landau, "Food Allergies Make Kids a Target of Bullies," CNN.com, September 28, 2010, http://www.cnn.com/2010 /HEALTH/09/28/food.allergy.bullying/index.html?eref=mrs s_igoogle_cnn.

ACKNOWLEDGMENTS

MANY PEOPLE HELPED EDEN WHEN he needed it most. Among them are Anna Nowak-Wegrzyn, Monique Bureau, Dana Fern, Russell Cohen, Madeline Dubin Strong, Marjorie Becker-Lewin, Susan Slesinger, Barbara Blum, and Mark Nesselson. Thank you to the many other medical professionals who gave us their time and attention along the way.

I'm forever grateful to everyone who helped me to write my first book: Amy Silverstein kindly pointed out a way. Then, my agent, Rebecca Gradinger, read and understood the story within my bulging manuscript. It was my good fortune for Zach Schisgal, my editor, to jump in as he did. Kathy Franklin offered her ongoing "support" and discretion. And Henry and Paul Ehrlich provided the good word when called upon. At Sterling Publishing, thank you to everyone who advanced this book, including Carlo DeVito, Scott Amerman, Rachel Maloney, and Leigh Ann Ambrosi.

Also my thanks go to my readers: Christopher Schelling, who gave me my first notes when he had no reason to take me seriously; Debbie Spurlock, who read it all just to do it; Julie Wang, Dominick Masiello, and Russell Cohen, who stepped in with their special expertise; and my friends and family who read the bits and pieces along the way (I hope it was worth the wait). Mom—your patience touched me. And Dad—you were my first fan club of one.

Finally, much love to Rob Wilder for telling me that I really could write this book, and to my husband for reminding me to believe him.

INDEX